Praise for Frank Wildman:

"There are ways that will lead you to a more active, healthy and safer life and you will feel, look and act younger. One of the best ways to do this is to read *Change Your Age* and follow the advice of Dr. Frank Wildman. He is a master teacher of Feldenkrais and many forms of vital movement therapy. I can highly recommend this book to all who wish to improve their well-being."

> —*Paul Davidson, MD, internist and rheumatologist and author of the best-selling* Chronic Muscle Pain Syndrome

"Dr. Wildman's Change Your Age Program comes from over 30 years of experience with people, bodies and ideas. He has combined insights from movement studies and neurophysiology to create a program that can enable and allow anyone of any age to improve their ability to move, think, act and feel."

> —*Sanford Rosenberg, PhD, psychologist and president of Media Research Associates*

"Frank Wildman hands down and hands on to us the richness and complexity of the Method directly from its founder, Moshe Feldenkrais."

> —*Michael McClure, Obie Award–winning playwright, poet and author of* The Beard *and* Scratching the Beat Surface

"Frank is one of those rare people who has both the gift to clearly understand the complex principles behind his work and the gift to communicate that work in a simple and intimate way."

> —*Jader Tolja, MD, professor at the University of Milan*

"Frank's teaching is totally inspirational. This is really about teaching and educating the person, instead of forcing someone through an exercise by repetition of a movement. As an instructor, it has given me another vantage point and a whole other vocabulary to communicate with my students. It has made my work exciting again!"

> —*Kathryn Ross-Nash, founding president of the Pilates Guild*

"Frank Wildman's enthusiasm for the work and dedication to its value in enhancing the human condition has led him to introduce the material to groups of health professionals nationally and internationally. He has a clear image of how a program can be most effective and combines this with a flair for light-hearted showmanship."

—*John B. Chester, MD, former director of pain services at Salem Hospital Regional Rehabilitation Center*

Frank Wildman's Change Your Age Program is a pleasure. Thousands of people could regain and enjoy the mobility they had when they were much younger. Read this book and do it.

—*Anna Halprin, post-modern dance and theatre pioneer*

I've experienced how you really can change your age several times with great pleasure. These movement routines are well thought out and give you plenty of time to stop, reflect, and repeat. I was particularly struck by Frank Wildman's perspective on how we can change habits that diminish our potential and bedevil aspects of our aging.

—*Brooks Adams, art critic and contributing editor,* Art in America

Frank Wildman is an exceptionally stimulating, generous, and knowledgeable teacher. He has a unique way of clarifying the relationship of the Feldenkrais Method to contemporary intellectual and scientific trends.

—*Yvan Joly, Feldenkrais trainer and psychologist*

CHANGE YOUR AGE

CHANGE YOUR AGE

USING YOUR BODY AND BRAIN TO FEEL YOUNGER, STRONGER, AND MORE FIT

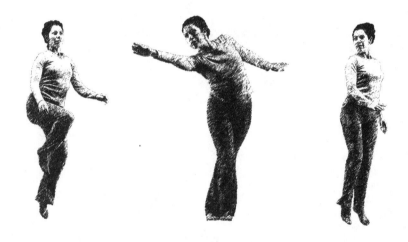

FRANK WILDMAN, CFT, PhD

Da Capo
∞
LIFE
LONG

A Member of the Perseus Books Group

Copyright © 2010 by Frank Wildman, CFT, PhD
Photos by R. J. Muna

Designed by Trish Wilkinson
Set in 11.5 point Goudy by the Perseus Books Group

Cataloging-in-Publication data for this book is available from the Library of Congress.

First Da Capo Press edition 2010
ISBN 978-0-7382-1363-7

Published by Da Capo Press
A Member of the Perseus Books Group
www.dacapopress.com

Note: The information in this book is true and complete to the best of our knowledge. This book is intended only as an informative guide for those wishing to know more about health issues. In no way is this book intended to replace, countermand, or conflict with the advice given to you by your own physician. The ultimate decision concerning care should be made between you and your doctor. We strongly recommend that you follow his or her advice. Information in this book is general and is offered with no guarantees on the part of the author or Da Capo Press. The author and publisher disclaim all liability in connection with the use of this book. The names and identifying details of people associated with events described in this book have been changed. Any similarity to actual persons is coincidental.

Da Capo Press books are available at special discounts for bulk purchases in the United States by corporations, institutions, and other organizations. For more information, please contact the Special Markets Department at the Perseus Books Group, 2300 Chestnut Street, Suite 200, Philadelphia, PA 19103, or call (800) 810-4145 extension 5000, or e-mail special.markets@perseusbooks.com.

10 9 8 7 6 5 4 3 2 1

To Beryl Kennedy, my student, friend, and mentor, who was doing clown dives at the age of 85; and to all the people who studied with me across this planet for so many years, and who proved to me that they could change their age, and demonstrated that the promises made in this book can be fulfilled.

CONTENTS

FOREWORD

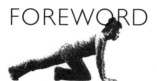

AGING ISN'T WHAT IT USED TO BE—BUT IT'S NOT YET WHAT IT COULD BE

by Ken Dychtwald, PhD

IN AN ancient Greek fable, Eos, the beautiful goddess of the dawn, falls deeply in love with the warrior Tithonus. Distraught over his mortality, she goes to Zeus's chamber to request a special favor: She wants to love Tithonus until the end of time and begs Zeus to grant her lover immortality. "Are you certain that is what you want for him?" Zeus challenges. "Yes," Eos responds.

As Eos leaves Zeus's chamber she realizes in shock that she forgot to ask that Tithonus also remain eternally young and healthy. With each passing year, she looks on with horror as he grows older and sicker. As the decades pass, the once-proud warrior is reduced to a collection of pained and increasingly fragile bones—yet continues to live forever.

This is a fitting allegory for what many of us are struggling with today—unhealthy aging. During the 20th century, we did an excellent job of eliminating many of the life-threatening diseases of youth. Childbirth, once a major cause of premature death, has by and large become healthier and safer.

The effect of these improvements is that more of us are living longer—but not necessarily healthier.

When we're young, we tend to take our health for granted. Then, when we reach our forties or fifties, we begin to notice that there are some changes going on, and we start to take things much more seriously. As we look at our own moms and dads, we can see the outcomes of how things turn out when people do or don't take the best care of themselves.

Luckily, many of my generation, the baby boomer generation, have begun changing our culture's perceptions of aging by creating healthy, active lifestyles. However, there is still a missing link in our perception of aging that has not been addressed: the mysteries of moving youthfully.

For nearly 40 years, I have been a student of the field of wellness and have written extensively about health, aging, and longevity. As I've traveled the world, I've encountered numerous enthusiastic practitioners, but only a handful of great teachers who were truly innovative. I have witnessed countless approaches to vitality and rejuvenation, but only a few that actually seem to work.

I wrote my first book, *Bodymind*, in the early 1970s, and during that time I had the good fortune of observing and experiencing Frank Wildman and his brilliant work. To this day, I remain absolutely dazzled by his nearly unrivaled knowledge of the workings of the body and mind, his ingenious therapeutic talents, and his masterful teaching style.

Dr. Wildman believes that the mind and body are intimately connected—like dancing partners. He teaches that our bodies are constantly being shaped and reshaped by the moves we make—or do not make. As we grow up, we learn to walk, eat, sleep, dance, make love, and think in certain ways. As we mature, unfortunately, we often move less, become creatures of our own habits, and stop learning to move in new ways. In response, our neuromuscular development diminishes, and we find ourselves with a growing legion of aches and pains, rigidities, limits, and other unpleasant manifestations of aging and dis-ease.

And so we're fortunate that Frank Wildman has distilled the lessons of his lifetime into a powerful, easy-to-follow new system for all of us. *Change Your Age* is a book for now and for the future. In the recent past, people didn't expect to move so well by the time they reached their forties and fifties. And lots of people didn't expect to be moving much at all by the time they reached their sixties and seventies.

This massive change in expectations and realities about our mobility could be called "the Movement Movement." Frank Wildman has been one of the world's foremost visionaries and leaders of this movement, bringing his skills with the Feldenkrais Method®, somatic psychology, and dance and movement arts to thousands of people in this country and abroad.

The Change Your Age Program presents an entirely new way of thinking about how we use our bodies and minds, and I believe it has the potential to revolutionize what we think of as the future of exercise. We can surely continue to strive for stronger muscles, but we also have to work for a stronger brain and a more clever and resilient body.

Change Your Age is the first movement-oriented program that intentionally arranges cognitive challenges while you move. This book contains much more than an exercise program. It's a way to help each of us feel the coordination of our minds and bodies in ways we have not previously considered. Through this process, we come to more fully understand how our bodies and minds are integrated while learning to feel and function so much better.

I have seen Frank Wildman teach 45-year-olds to move like 30-year-olds. Although that might not seem like much, if you're 50 or 55 and could be handed back 10 to 15 years of your movement abilities, you might assume it to be an act of God. If you are a well-functioning 70-year-old, you might find yourself lusting for the mobility of a 50-year-old. In fact, Dr. Wildman's movement programs have helped many middle-aged men and women achieve a dexterity and agility that they haven't had since they were teenagers. And therein lies the attraction of his remarkable system. It's not a tedious set of exercises or a no-pain-no-gain collection of strenuous workouts. It's an ingenious, enjoyable approach to retraining your bodymind to feel and function as though it were young again.

What I find particularly intelligent about Dr. Wildman's approach is that he doesn't evoke anything supernatural, but he is fiercely focused on your capacity to learn new and easier ways of moving.

When you finish these lessons, you'll find yourself feeling more limber and free of old aches and pains. Your carriage, posture, and the quality of your movement will seem more vigorous, more energized—even more youthful.

And so take a deep breath, turn the page, and get ready to change your age!

Ken Dychtwald, PhD
psychologist, gerontologist, and author of Bodymind, Healthy Aging,
The Keys to a High-Performance Lifestyle, Age Power, *and* With Purpose

INTRODUCTION

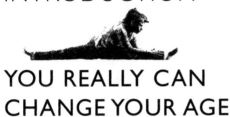

YOU REALLY CAN
CHANGE YOUR AGE

Through the first years of life, we organize our entire system in a direction which will forever after guide us in that direction. We end up being restricted, we don't do music, we don't do other things. What is more important, we find ourselves capable of doing only those things that we already know.

—Moshe Feldenkrais, DSc, San Francisco, 1977

WHAT MAKES a person old? Some people think it's wrinkles; others say it's stodgy attitudes. But, really, the culprit is our habits. When we unlearn old habits and create new ones, we make our bodies and minds younger, stronger, and more flexible. In essence, we create a more youthful and intelligent body at any age.

Unlike other members of the animal kingdom, as humans, we only gradually learn how to control our bodies. To survive as infants and children, we must learn to lift our heads, push up our chests, sit, crawl, walk, jump, skip, and run. Once we learn these increasingly complex movements, we stop the learning process, and our movements become habituated, often in ways that put stress on our bodies or that become rigidified and locked over time. We're left with a lifetime of habits—from how we swing a tennis racket or sit at the keyboard to how we move when we cook a gourmet meal—that can become harmful to our bodies. The good news is that we can learn new habits that make our bodies and minds more agile and more fit.

The easy-to-learn exercises and sequences in this book will help you break away from physically limiting habits and steer you toward feeling as you ordinarily would at your best—and perhaps, youngest—moments. With the Change Your Age Program, you will move beyond the idea of doing exercises the "right" way or measuring how well you're doing by looking at yourself in the mirror and instead return to moving as you did when you were younger.

Although exercise and movement in general can feel good and be considered health-related, not many people make the same connection between exercise and their brain. Using the principles of neuroscience, you can learn to guide your body internally in order to discover new sensations, a new and wider range of movement, and new techniques for coordinating your movements for ease and efficiency. You will engage your whole body and your brain in simple but powerful movement sequences that can actually re-groove your brain's neuropathways so that you will begin to move in healthier, stronger, more coordinated, and even more graceful ways. These exercises are adaptable to you and your exact needs. The results you see in your heightened sense of vitality and youthfulness will attest to their effectiveness.

One of the best ways to reverse the all-too-common effects of aging is to move well and use your whole body. You can have a spring in your step, an air of grace, and stability and ease of movement at any age. What it means to be 50 today—how you function, what you are able to achieve, your life expectations, and your appearance—is very different from just 50 years ago. Much has been learned in recent years about the process of optimal aging. The discovery that movement and exercise regulate neurogenesis—that is, the production of new neurons in the adult brain—has been the surprising news that fundamentally changes our view on how physical activity affects the brain.[1]

Previously, it was thought that we never grow new neurons. Throughout life, this theory went, we maintain whatever number we were born with except for those that die in our heads—and thus end up with fewer and fewer neurons. A bleak view. This understanding was challenged, however, by the experience of people with serious traumatic injuries who not only could learn new things but could also learn to move, think, and speak even better than they did before the damaging incident. What was happening? New technology now allows us to watch nerves grow and to watch nerve fibers "rewiring" and "networking" with each other as new motor skills are learned and practiced. The brain has proven to be more "plastic" and is now regarded as capable of changing its function and interior forms. Neurons regenerate until the day you die! An old dog *can* learn new tricks.

We also know through extensive research that continued learning and exercise in middle age and beyond increases longevity[2] and has benefits for both overall health and cognitive function, especially in later life.[3] Your behavior at age 50 has an impact on how you feel at age 80. High-density brain analyses show that voluntary exercise can increase brain growth factors that stimulate the generation of neurons, increase resistance to brain insult, and improve learning and mental performance.[4] Intelligent exercise could provide a simple means to maintain brain function and promote brain plasticity and neurogenesis.[5] Exercise combined with cognitively stimulating movements results in optimal aging.

The Change Your Age Program is based on the ability of our brains to grow, function, and improve through practice and on the fact that we can improve with age. We cannot achieve greater quality of movement by stretching or strengthening muscle groups alone. Coordinating our bodies and brains, however, will improve how we move and alter many of the signs of aging.

In this program, you'll have an opportunity to feel, think, and move simultaneously. You'll be using your brain to experience your body as a mystery being revealed to you, and you'll be using your body to learn new movements and new feelings that are revealed to your brain. As you learn new qualities of movement, you'll gain not only a deeper sense of yourself but a richer connection between your brain and your body.

The fact is that our brain is our core, and through our neural pathways it operates every part of the body. It's easy to think of the brain as a super-smart tool that tells us what to say, where to go, what to do, what to think, and what to feel. But that's not the whole story.

Although the brain does send signals throughout the body, it also receives signals that give us important information. If we learn how to listen better to what our bodies are telling us, we can also learn to pay attention to the inside of our own bodies and receive these signals as vital and important information. For example, in the places where we're tight and tense or loose and fit, where we're injured and in pain or flooded with pleasure, we can discover the connection between our minds and bodies. We can begin to move more easily and to feel stronger and more confident about who we are.

The brain is the essential component that is largely missing from all other workout and body movement programs. We often move and exercise as if we didn't have one. However, changes in behavior can change the way we age. This program emphasizes changing the quality of your body's movement and your brain's involvement in that movement. By the time you complete the exercises in this book, you'll have more poise in your posture and more confidence in your step, and you will find yourself looking and feeling younger.

● ● ●

I WAS a young performing artist and choreographer, studying psychology, aging, and physical therapies, when I met Moshe Feldenkrais, the creator of the Feldenkrais Method®. He had a whole new approach to the body, the mind, and movement that bridged the physical and mental domains in a way that was unlike any other discipline I had studied or practiced. At the center of the Feldenkrais Method® are lessons that explore developmental movements and access the power and plasticity of the central nervous system to improve human function by increasing self-awareness in movement.

I became Dr. Feldenkrais's first North American student and apprenticed with the great movement scientist over a period of ten years while continuing my graduate studies in biology and psychology with a specialty in movement sciences. I became the first educational director of Feldenkrais practitioner trainings after his death in 1984. Then I created Feldenkrais professional training programs worldwide, helping hundreds of people develop successful careers in a variety of fields, from sports medicine to physical therapy to the arts.

For over 30 years, I have also applied these ideas in clinical settings, working one on one and with groups to address every possible kind of physical limitation and to enhance and develop the mind-body connection. With my background in the sciences, I was able to introduce the Feldenkrais Method in medical settings, often to groups that included psychologists, orthopedists, and physical therapists.

I developed the first movement education program for senior citizens at the University of California, which led to "Improving with Age," a project of training teachers and therapists in a radically different approach to working with older adults in an attempt to change the concept of exercise. In that program, I addressed the movement difficulties of older adults, which got me thinking about how older adults could avoid these problems in the first place.

What I came to see was that, if middle-aged adults readjusted their habits, they could enter their later years with a much sounder approach to their movements. I began training people to discover their own myth of aging and to see how that myth could limit them for the rest of their life. Taking clients from "where they are now" and teaching them how to move more effectively, I was able to help them access their own potential peak performance.

Drawing from over 30 years of my experience, the Change Your Age Program developed for this book is specifically suited to the needs of a generation of midlife baby boomers who are seeking lifelong fitness, not for reasons having to do with physique or vanity, but for wellness.

● ● ●

THE CHANGE Your Age Program includes several body-mind assessment tools and over 30 movement lessons, sequenced according to the five core positions of human movement—lying down, sitting, kneeling, crouching, and standing.

- First, Chapter 1 will help you consider what might be helpful or harmful in your current exercise program and discusses what might be missing from your workout.
- Next, Chapter 2 will give you the tools to assess the state of your body so that you can better understand how to create your dream body.
- In Chapter 2, you will also have the chance to take the Change Your Age Mobility Survey to get a sense of your areas of strength and the areas where you have room for improvement. Please visit our website (www.changeyourage.net) to take a more comprehensive survey and get your Change Your Age Mobility Index score. You can also sign up for our newsletter and get more helpful information on how to change your age.
- In Chapter 3, you will learn several movement lessons for each of the five core positions of lying, sitting, kneeling, crouching, and standing, as well as more advanced variations, to release, extend, strengthen, and heal your body.
- In Chapters 4 and 5, once you have become familiar with each movement sequence, you will be able to create your own routines to meet your individual needs and address the challenges you face with everyday movement and the activities you love. You will be able to combine what you learn in the Change Your Age Program with any meditation or exercise routines that you enjoy.

After just a couple of weeks of using the program, you will begin to experience a "younger" body and a "younger" mind, as I've seen with many of my clients. I've discovered how to keep my clients, my students, and myself more youthful as we age. Now I want to share this knowledge and this program with you.

But before we begin, you need to *believe* that you can change your age.

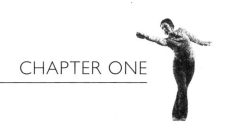

CHAPTER ONE

HOW TO ASSESS YOUR CURRENT EXERCISE PROGRAM

Is Your Current Exercise Routine Helping or Harming You?

THE MORE you move, the better off you are. You can build a better heart, and recent research shows that you can build a better brain. You can build stronger bones, joints, ligaments, tendons, and muscles. Your blood flow improves, which enables the liquids in your body to circulate more effectively. All of these things are keys to a younger, stronger body.

But there is a dilemma. What if you have been exercising but you are hurting or feel stiff and have to work out the kinks every day? What if the kind of movement you're doing will become more difficult as you age?

We are familiar with the idea that certain habits are bad for our health or might contribute to premature aging. Habits such as smoking, overeating, overdrinking, or a complete lack of exercise are often mentioned as factors that contribute to the aging process, but we don't often think about the impact of our movement habits—how we hold tension in our neck or lower back, how inefficiently we breathe, how we shovel snow, or even how we run or do yoga. Over our lifetimes, these movement habits can contribute to aging just as dramatically. How many people have picked up a snow shovel to clean the driveway only to be laid up that night with a bad back? Or gone to the gym after a period of inactivity only to be so sore the next day that they couldn't continue? How many people, just sitting rigidly at a desk all day, discover that their shoulders have become permanently hunched?

Habits are seductive. We like to think that we could keep exercising or playing sports and maintain all of our old habits. The dilemma is that old habits can become dangerous to our joints by overstressing ligaments and causing strains, injuries, and tears in our muscles.

In fact, exercise could be a dangerous thing.

When we exercise, we become inflamed and overheated. The aftereffects can be either uplifting and energizing or fatiguing and uninspiring. This all depends on who you are and how you move.

We do have a saving grace: If we exercise with awareness, we can prevent most injuries and improve our movement habits and the elegance of our posture and bearing.

Your main muscle, the brain, is the core of your strength, stability, motivation, and self-awareness. Your muscles, sensations, and ability to move would be impossible without your brain. If you want to keep improving as you age, vigorous, routine exercise will not be as effective as using your brain to learn how to move in new ways, just as you did when you were a child.

As humans, we enjoy complexity and variety, and we can exercise in ways similar to how we "exercised" when we were children and, before that, infants.

Can you imagine tying wrist and ankle weights around an infant so that he becomes stronger? Or stretching a baby's body into different positions to make her more flexible? This is the way we start to treat ourselves by the time we are in our late teens. Learning to become an adult often means learning to perform dull, repetitive routines instead of holding on to the active curiosity and exploratory movements of our youth.

Eventually we don't need to keep exploring certain basic movements—we "just do it." But a critically important feature of improving your functional mobility and changing your age is to return to those more youthful exploratory movements.

No matter what your level of fitness is, or your current exercise routine, your concerns about injuries, pain, or restricted movement, or your overall sense of wellness or fatigue, the Change Your Age Program can make you feel younger, more graceful, more flexible, more coordinated, and more at ease. By practicing movements that make you feel younger, you can regain the ease you felt 10 or 15 years ago. This chapter discusses the dangers of exercise and the tendencies toward bad movement that many common exercise programs encourage; I'll help you discover whether your current routine is actually *aging* you. We explore things you can do to establish new and more vital habits. You will learn how to improve your body awareness and how to harness that awareness as a tool to transform your functional age. You will also return to learning as you once did as a child, using exploratory movement.

● ● ●

THE DANGERS OF EXERCISE: OVERSTRESSING

Many people believe that exercise is not really good for them unless they feel hyperstimulated or have some background fatigue, which they often identify as relaxing because they have worn out their muscles. Overexercising and the stresses that ensue lead to metabolic changes from the creation of more free radicals that age all our cells. We also get micro-tears in our connective tissues and micro-fractures in our skeletons, which contribute to lost mobility over time and can lead to premature aging.

Most people can withstand substantial injuries early in their life and make remarkable comebacks with relatively short recovery times. As we get older, it becomes more important to avoid injuries, because it is more difficult to heal and an injury can have ramifications beyond the ability to do a workout routine. For example, sustaining an injury to your knee that prevents you from getting up and down from the floor easily or climbing your stairs can become a significant life-changing event if it causes long-term pain that affects your job, your relationships, and even your living quarters. I had a client who ran and rock-climbed regularly, but then seriously injured his knee. Although he continued to do the activities that were familiar and enjoyable to him for a while, eventually he couldn't even make it up the stairs. By learning some of the movements in the Change Your Age Program, he was able to go up and down stairs without pain and then return to the activities he enjoyed.

Overstressing during exercise can create additional stresses to the joints and ligaments of the body. Your ligaments connect one bone to another and connect your skeleton together. If you had no muscles or tendons (which connect your muscles to your bones), you would still be held together by your ligaments. Forceful movement done too frequently has an effect on a ligament similar to taking a fresh, taut rubber band and pulling it apart and together repeatedly or pulling the band apart to its limit and keeping it there for too long. The band, like your ligaments, loses elasticity, and a ligament with less elasticity can weaken the bone-to-bone connections in your body.

In my work, I see highly skilled athletes, weekend athletes, and sports enthusiasts as well as well-renowned dance teachers and yoga instructors. Many of them come to me because of injuries they have sustained doing their favorite activities.

Many yoga teachers have stretched for too long or too far and, slowly, lengthened their ligaments. When we stretch too much, our ligaments become loose so our joints become too loose and they lose their stability. This unstable joint condition, known as hypermobility, arises from moving the joint too far and too often.

Similarly, runners, as they get older, find themselves getting tight in the calves and hamstrings, developing knee injuries, and then having to do a lot of stretching to help defray the feeling of tightness.

"Boomeritis," named in 1999 by Dr. Nicholas A. DiNubile, an orthopedic surgeon at the Hospital of the University of Pennsylvania, is a national phenomenon witnessed by many physicians. Their baby boomer patients have returned to exercising, but they are exercising in the only way they're familiar with, which is the exercise they knew in their twenties and thirties. The *-itis* in boomeritis refers to the mass inflammation of muscles, tendons, and joints that usually results in the breakdown of muscles and the supporting organs of the body, like the heart and kidneys, which are necessary to process the full metabolic and physiological effects of exercise on the body. Boomeritis can be completely avoided, however, by starting slower, using less force, and, if you're following the exercise instructions of a personal trainer, listening only to someone who is trained in working with older adults. You'll find one of the best ways to return to moving your body in the slow, inventive, and unusual movements of Chapter 3.

Here are four quick questions to help you assess whether overstressing is a problem in your exercise routines:

- Do you exercise beyond the point of pain and stress?
- Do you feel that you have not exercised enough if you don't feel pain?
- While you exercise, do you feel yourself straining?
- How do you feel the next day?

THE LIMITS OF LEARNING BY IMITATION

Although it is better to move your body than not, you need to have an increased awareness of how you move in order to prevent injuries. Moving well isn't good enough without knowing *how* you move, a point not often stressed in typical workout routines.

Knowing *why* you have an injury or a pain is not so helpful. However, knowing *how* you move your body, arrange your posture, or perform repeated actions that created or contributed to your pain or injury is a valuable thing to know. Knowing why you're uncoordinated might not help you to be more coordinated, but learning how to move differently will address the situation directly. Knowing *why* might not be useful to you; knowing *how* is a physical tool you can acquire and use.

You can become skilled at dance or sports but have no idea how you acquired that skill. (This is a primary reason why highly skilled professionals often cannot teach others.) It may be that you have very limited body awareness, but that you can mimic movement very well. Most people learn to move by visual imitation—that is, by watching other people's movements and imitating them. This is the way classes are taught in dance, theater, and sports. Even social interactions usually involve visual imitation.

Learning by visual imitation does not require that we advance our body awareness; instead, it requires that we perform what we already know how to do, usually by trying to conform our bodies to the instructor's body. That's why many people start learning very quickly; their lack of body awareness, however, makes them unable to improve continuously. Visually, they can see what to do, and their body can imitate and mimic very well, but this capacity to mimic does not tell them how they learned the movement. We can perform a movement through imitation if our body already understands how to do it. If our body doesn't already know how to do a movement, we can't progress or improve beyond that point without improving our body awareness.

In the Change Your Age Program, you will find yourself developing your body awareness by learning *how* to do the movements. Many of the movements will not resemble familiar actions. The novelty of the movements will stimulate your brain to forge new connections. Without novelty, we reinforce the same habits.

Ask yourself the following questions as they relate to your current exercise routine.

- Is it difficult for me to learn new movement skills?
- Can I easily teach others new ways to move?
- Do new challenges in movement make you feel excited or anxious?

COMPETING WITH YOURSELF

Whether you run, work with weights, do yoga, or engage in sports like tennis, golf, basketball, soccer, swimming, or skiing, you can be subject to repetitive stress injuries. As you get older, more stress injuries can arise from a competition with yourself.

The drive that leads to most injuries is the drive to outdo yourself. Rather than doing exercise slowly, easily, and gradually, people adopt the credo "no pain, no gain" and try to stretch the farthest they can, in competition either with others or with themselves. A doctor might say that for the health of your heart, you should get off the couch and lose weight, starting by exercising 30 minutes a day, three times a week. But some people get on machines at the gym and go crazy. They think that, if 30 minutes is good, 40 minutes would be better, 50 minutes would be even better, and 60 minutes would be best. They apply the same attitude to speed and slope: Faster and steeper is better. But that is not the case: When you exercise harder, you also stress your body more. People competing hard against themselves get stronger muscles, but there is a trade-off between how hard you exercise and how stressed your body becomes.

Additionally, we're all caught up in perceptions of age that are based on physical appearance. This is what drives so many people to extend themselves in unhealthy ways by striving for washboard abs, tight triceps, the perfect butt.

Instead of "no pain, no gain," the attitude should be "no pain, all gain in the brain."

In considering whether or not competing with yourself has become too much of a problem with your current exercise habits, ask yourself these questions:

- Do I try to outdo myself with each workout?
- Do I measure my success only by achieving extremes?
- Could I assess myself by the sensual pleasure a workout gives me?

QUANTITY VERSUS QUALITY

The study of human motion—quantifying the human body by measuring how much and how many times people can move—emerged as the industrial age took hold and virtually all bodies began to move in harmony with assembly lines and other machinery or equipment.

At this time, exercise as a formal discipline began to be studied as something quantifiable. Whether health-related or work-related, the key issues became how much, how many times, how far, how fast, how big, and how strong.

As research into the human body and exercise continued, it became more and more necessary for researchers to focus their studies on the quantification of movement. The question of how far or how long a person should run was researched endlessly, but *how* a person runs—the quality of the running—was not investigated. When we watch wide receivers on football teams who are famously graceful; or sleek, long-limbed guards in the NBA; or runners whose stride is beautifully smooth; the quality of their movement or their grace may attract our attention and capture our hearts. But today many people don't value the same grace of movement in their own exercise: They focus on the quantity of their movement ("How far did I walk?" "Did I exercise enough?") rather than the quality.

Aiming to achieve goals that are easy to quantify can create excessive tension in the effort to achieve those goals, which ends up being counterproductive. In the Change Your Age Program, I won't emphasize the number of repetitions you need to do, but rather the quality of your movements and your awareness of them. Evaluate the role that quantity and quality of motion play in your current exercise routines.

- Are measurable quantities—repetitions, time, weight, speed—more important to you than your quality of motion?
- Can you assess your typical workout's success to include your gracefulness in performing the movement?
- When you move, do you feel you move more like a machine or an animal? What image of a graceful animal could you bring to your workout?

THE PATH OF MOST RESISTANCE

Many forms of exercise use increasing resistance as the only path to building strength. Thousands of repetitions against greater and greater resistance eventually increases the strength and size of our muscles.

Some people lift weights or spend hours on machines that exercise the same muscle group in the same fashion over and over again. The very feeling of intramuscular stress or tired muscles is considered an indication of a good workout.

This approach, however, can result in more problems than benefits: When our muscles can contract more powerfully, any existing muscular-skeletal imbalance or faulty movement habit becomes exaggerated and am-plified. If you haven't learned to lift properly, you are at greater risk for stress-related pain and damage to your ligaments and tendons with strong muscles than with weak ones. If you use too much effort in getting up, stand-ing, running, and so on, stronger muscles only mask the problem. These sorts of ineffective movement habits overwork certain muscles and joints while neglecting or ignoring the use of others, thus leading to a limited range of movement and gross inefficiency. The brain might be engaging far more muscle cells to perform simple activities like sitting in a chair than are neces-sary to perform the action required.

For example, some people can sit in a chair engaging 20 percent or more of the muscle fibers in their back, while other people can sit in the same posture using as little as 2 percent of these brain-to-muscle connections (called motor units). This disparity in effort obviously leads to tremendous differences in how long people can sit comfortably without compressing their spine and overworking their back muscles.

In the long run, limitations in awareness and coordination can lead to se-vere physical difficulties and prematurely age us. Parts of our articulations or joints can fill with fibrous tissues, especially between vertebrae, where there is little movement in general. Ligaments shorten or become hyper-elastic. Some muscle fibers become too strong, while others in the same muscle group atrophy. In time, deformation sets in. Without body awareness, we ex-ercise our worst habits.

Strength is not simply a function of our muscles. We can strengthen all of our muscles, but if we don't use our brain to improve their organization and coordination, we do not significantly improve our posture, deftness, perfor-mance, or stability.

Consider the amount of resistance in your current exercise routine.

- Does your exercise routine value strength over mobility or flexibility?
- Do you pay attention to your posture while either doing resistance ex-ercises or running and cycling?

WORK VERSUS EFFORT

A major goal in life could be to accomplish the same amount of work with less effort. The distinction between work and the amount of effort required to produce the work needs to be felt in our body. Lifting your weight out of a chair and lifting your handbag from the floor are both actions that involve measurable amounts of work depending on your weight and on what's in the handbag. The amount of effort required to get out of a chair or to lift a handbag can vary from person to person tremendously. Some people strain, hold their breath, and grunt when picking up almost anything, while others are so efficient and relaxed while performing the same work that they display little effort.

In all movements, groups of agonist muscles and antagonist muscles are at work. Agonist muscles are the primary muscles—the ones doing the contracting—in movement. When you lift something in front of yourself with your arms, the biceps are the main actors, the agonist muscles. Antagonist muscles oppose the agonists. They are the muscle fibers on the other side of the joint, and they work opposite to the action. When lifting something in front of yourself with your arms, the triceps are the antagonists.

If you operate with 10 percent of the antagonists opposing the action of the agonists, your muscles have to work harder and exert more effort, owing to this internal resistance. You may not feel the tug-of-war between the muscle groups, how hard your antagonist muscle groups are contradicting your intended direction of motion. Ideally, you want to reduce the internal resistance of your antagonist muscles so that more force can be available for your daily actions through your agonist muscles.

If you lack the ability to reduce your internal resistance, you will always feel the need to be stronger and will feel less effective at exerting mechanical force on the outside world, such as when you lift objects, open doors, climb stairs, or dance.

Injuries and the resulting pain often create neuromuscular inefficiency that increases resistance in the area that hurts. One of the best strategies is to learn to move the painful area easily, lightly, and slowly so that the brain can learn comfort in relation to the intended movement. Doing less is actually more! This is one goal of the lessons of the Change Your Age Program.

You could race through the entire Change Your Age Program, get a workout, build up a sweat, and feel quite good in that familiar way, maybe even proud of yourself for having accomplished all of the movements quickly. However, if you never learn to do these movements slowly and comfortably, if you do not decrease your internal resistance, and if you do not increase your *felt sense* of the movements—your body awareness—then you will finish the program having learned absolutely nothing. Your brain will probably make no changes, and so your body, as if it had no brain, will get no benefit from the program beyond the one workout.

Consider the amount of effort required to accomplish your usual workout routine as well as ordinary activities of daily life like walking up stairs and carrying groceries from the car.

- Do you catch yourself straining or grunting to accomplish a task?
- Can you feel your antagonist muscles at work? For example, do you feel strain in your triceps when you are using your biceps to lift something?
- Pick several of your normal daily activities and think about how much work is required to carry them out. Can you imagine performing the same amount of work doing these activities with less effort?

● ● ●

CREATING MORE VITAL HABITS

So far, I have asked you to reflect on whether you are susceptible to any of the dangers of exercise described here. Now I'd like to introduce you to some possibly unfamiliar movement concepts that are central to the Change Your Age Program. These ideas can help you mitigate the dangers and damaging habits of your current exercise routine by helping you develop a sensory tool that enables you to feel what you are doing and to discern what might be dangerous or simply too difficult for you. With this sensory tool, called human awareness, you'll fall away from dull, repetitive, and harmful routines and engage in more youthful movement.

BODY AWARENESS:
THE KEY TO INJURY PREVENTION

The more aware you are of your body, the more you can avoid injuries. Body awareness should never be considered an add-on to an exercise routine, but rather the foundation. Nothing will protect your back or your knees more than having the body awareness to know how to move in a protective manner. Strong but uninformed and unaware muscles are not helpful to your joints.

We need our brains to understand our limits when we exercise so that we don't strain our bodies into injury. It's our ideas about ourselves that lead us to overstress and overuse our bodies, but our brains can also provide us with the awareness of when it's time to stop.

Not allowing time for recovery from overexercising is one of the major sources of injury and pain. Overtraining is becoming a major issue for young athletes as more and more research points to the need for rest between exercise sessions. This becomes more true as we get older. When you feel the inflammatory sore muscle effect of exercise or the achiness of your newly growing muscles, the actual growth and conditioning effects occur after the event itself, and mostly while you are sleeping. If you want to maximize the potential of your mind-body, dance and exercise in innovative ways and sleep for strength.

The State of the Body Scan, which is found in the next chapter, is a great first step in noticing and feeling more—like hearing better when you have your ears cleaned or finally getting the right glasses to make the blurriness disappear. You'll learn to have fuller proprioception.

Proprioception is your sixth sense. It refers to all the information that is poured into your brain from inside your body, telling you how you are sitting, standing, or lying and how you will need to move to get to the next position. Proprioception is what allows you to walk across a completely dark room by integrating your sense of balance with all the other input from inside your body. It is a major sense.

This sense allows you to scratch an itch on your knee in exactly the right spot, even in the dark or with your eyes closed. If people drink too much, some bodily control based on proprioception is hampered. Fatigue or simple sleepiness can also make this happen. When a police officer asks a driver to close his eyes and touch his nose, he is testing the person's proprioception.

These may seem like mundane examples of what this sense does for you, but without proprioception, you would be far more helpless than if you were blind or deaf or lacking a sense of smell or taste. You wouldn't be able to control your movements at all. You wouldn't be able to bring food to your mouth, tend to a wound, or move your body out of danger.

Strengthening the muscles of your body is a good thing, increasing your bone density is a great idea, and having the easy flexibility to perform daily tasks is useful. There are countless exercise programs to address issues of strength and flexibility.

But if you want to increase the quality of your motions—that is, the smoothness of your movements, the ease in your posture, the coordination of all the parts of your body acting as a whole—you need a program that develops your proprioception, your sense of the internal, your body awareness.

Improving body awareness is the key to change that leads to a more youthful body.

TUNE IN

Developing internal tools to help you notice changes gives you the chance to change your behavior in order to reduce pain and improve your ability to function.

The first step in developing these internal tools is to tune in to the signal. Tuning in to the signal requires that you turn down the noise, light, and effort so that you can notice the differences that you don't usually detect. When you do so, you will sense another body inside of yourself, and the experience is magical.

Once you learn how to tune in to the signals of your body, you can sense where you feel older inside and where you feel more youthful and then make changes to your movements accordingly to keep improving as you age. In

Chapter 2, you will be asked to observe your body and to apply this observation to your everyday life and current exercise routines.

My client Gary, a man in his fifties, is a great example of the dangers of exercise and the benefits of applying the concepts of increasing body awareness and exploratory learning. Gary was an avid skier and for much of his adult life had traveled throughout the world seeking the best slopes and the best snow. When he was younger, he had injured himself a couple of times, but he recovered and, of course, continued seeking snow.

Though he had not been injured again, he came to me with new pains in his back and a frozen shoulder, which had practically immobilized him and made him wonder whether he might have to stop skiing that season. His frozen shoulder was a result of his joint becoming unstable. Many people experience pain from exercises or sports because their brain can't organize the muscles close to the joint, which serve to stabilize the joint during any activity.

I worked with his balance, which is so important to maintain as we age. Gary had never realized the many differences between his left and right sides. He saw that he was using his right arm with the ski poles very differently than the way he used his left arm. He knew he was better able to turn on his skis to one side but didn't understand why— he didn't understand how his body parts turned differently or balanced differently on one side compared to another.

Gary's shoulder injury was a complete mystery to him, since no incident had occurred that would have particularly aggravated his right shoulder. I helped him feel, from the inside, how he was moving his trunk. Away from the stress of both skiing and his off-season exercising, he was able to sense much finer and subtler movements.

Once Gary learned how to tune in to the right signal, he had a much more refined sense of *how* he used his body on the left side, *how* he used it on the right side, and *how* he moved from left to right. Once he could sense more subtle movements and tensions in his body, Gary could then learn to alter those tensions, as well as the basic physical habits of a lifetime.

For him, this revelation was like magic. His frozen shoulder disappeared as he regained full use of it, and his back pain disappeared as well. Gary had learned that he was working his muscles with too much force in an attempt to ski the same way he did when he was young. No ski coaches had been able to help him because his problem was an "inside job." To celebrate solving that problem, Gary joined a team of his friends the next winter and was dropped by helicopter onto the Columbia ice fields.

● ● ●

EXPLORATORY MOVEMENT

An exploratory movement is a movement you perform when you don't know exactly what you are going to do so you have to think about it and feel your way through it. One example of exploratory movement is the kind of movement we all performed as babies trying to find where our hands, mouth, and feet were. Much more of your brain is used, and a far larger range of neurons are activated, when you're exploring a movement. As you keep practicing what you already know—that is, doing performatory movements—you use fewer new neuromuscular connections.

I call this combination of simultaneously thinking and feeling as you move "flinking," as a way to urge my students not to compartmentalize these mental and physical activities. As happened when you were a child, the greater the area of your brain that's involved in your movements, the more fit your brain becomes and the more it retains and generates new neural connections. The more you use your body awareness, the more you integrate the body and mind and the more proficient your movements and actions become.

For example, imagine that you are preparing to do a dead lift—lifting a weight off the floor until you are standing. If you are like most people, you have one way of performing this action and think that, if you made your muscles stronger, you could lift more weight. However, a completely different and healthier approach would be to explore how many ways you can coordinate your pelvis, legs, arms, and shoulders as well as your balance, timing, and breathing—in other words, your whole body—to lift the weight. This approach would make you not only stronger but better able to bend down and pick up anything, because you would have expanded your neuromuscular repertoire for bending over to pick things up.

The Change Your Age Program encourages the growth of your brain by having you use nonlinear movements like the ones you explored regularly when you were younger.

NONLINEAR MOVEMENT AND LEARNING

Many of us are trapped in a rigid way of learning with our current fitness routines. Some of us fixate on targeting specific muscle areas (to get that hard-body look, for example) or on specific joint actions (perhaps to perfect a tennis serve) instead of paying attention to how the whole system works in an integrated manner. Proprioceptive awareness can fade into the background and become irrelevant to the way we exercise. Without this awareness, we lose out on the important information it delivers that could help us avoid pain, stiffness, and injuries.

Additionally, exercise equipment is designed in a way to make bodies move in a machine-like fashion: on a single plane of action, up and down or side to side. The nature of exercise on these machines becomes linear movement, which is very different from the nonlinear ways in which we normally move—for example, as we reach for things that are a little off to the side, or twist our trunk to turn toward a friend while walking. In fact, many people with strong backs injure themselves and get incapacitating back spasms because they do a simple movement—such as retrieving a dropped dinner napkin at an angle and with a spinal twist—that they have never explored while exercising!

We rarely see twists, torques, and asymmetrical movements in exercise routines because, as people get older, they lose their ability to perform these kinds of movements. Older people who can spiral, twist, and move on strong diagonals always appear to be much younger than they are. Remember Tina Turner performing at her concerts when she was in her fifties? Or the Rolling Stones going on and on, performing nonlinear movements onstage at an age when most people have retired?

Because of this tendency to practice movements that target only partial areas of muscles and strengthen only partial areas of the bones, ligaments, and tendons, adults often engage not just a narrow area of their bodies but also only a narrow portion of their neurons. Their ability to learn is limited.

Infants and children, on the other hand, practice movement and learn in a very different way. Babies and young children exploring the environment reach and twist, shift and fall back. Those exploratory movements require the full use of the whole body, not just a good set of abs or a perfectly functioning shoulder joint.

As you age, it is crucial to return to moving like a child and learning like a child in this exploratory and nonlinear fashion. You don't need to avoid linear movement—in fact, many common daily activities are linear movements—but if you want to expand the range and repertoire of your movements and feel real pleasure and sensuality in your movements, you'll find it valuable to practice nonlinear and exploratory movements.

It really is possible to regain youth and vitality through body awareness and movement. You don't have to give up your exercise routines, but there are many valuable modifications you can make to help you get the most out of them.

As you begin to use Chapter 2's body awareness tools and then move on to Chapter 3's nonlinear exploratory movement program for adults, you will find yourself regaining years and vitality while discovering new ways to sense, think, and move.

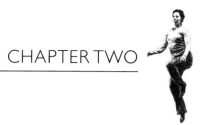

A STATE OF THE BODY REPORT

*How Is Your Body Today? How Do You
Want Your Body to Be Tomorrow?*

IN THIS chapter, you will learn a variety of new and easy ways to assess your "movement age," which you can use as a base to return to days, weeks, and months after starting the program. Some of these diagnostic tools are practical, while others are reflective; both kinds are unique assessment tools that will help you learn to increase your body awareness.

Machines can externally measure the condition of your body, but in this chapter I want you to become your own biofeedback device and internally sense the state of your body. You don't need expensive equipment; instead, all you need is your body, your mind, the floor, and your attention.

HIDDEN IN SLOW, SMALL MOVEMENTS— THE POTENTIAL FOR CHANGE

It is by paying attention that you can assess how young or old different parts of your body feel, determine the realistic and reasonable changes needed to make your movements more youthful, and measure your progress toward your goal of a more youthful self. Some of the changes required to reach your goal may be very small, but by quieting your environment and paying attention to your body, you can observe how these small changes lead to big adjustments.

You sense your environment and yourself in a variety of ways with five completely different types of senses: teleceptic, kinesthetic, proprioceptive, vestibular, and tactile.

Many of your senses are located primarily in your head and near your mouth: your eyes to see, your ears to hear, your nose to smell, and your mouth to taste. These are called *teleceptors*, meaning that they telescope external information from the environment, perhaps far from your body, so that you can see where you are going from a distance, hear a sound and know where it's coming from, smell whether you would enjoy a restaurant's food, or even distinguish friend from foe.

Your sense of taste is less *telescopic* because it's usually related to chewing and swallowing, actions that are not teleceptic; they are *kinesthetic* or internal senses. Chewing and swallowing are a passage from your teleceptic to your internal senses, which are often less valued and not always understood. They include all the sensations of your organs, from your heart beating, to your stomach growling and digesting, to your liver developing a stitch after intense exercise, to the pleasure experienced from sex.

The feedback of your contracting muscles, telling you how tight or relaxed they are, comes from your *proprioceptive* sense. Proprioception also tells you the position of your joints and where your body parts are in space.

The *vestibular* system is located inside the inner ear and gives you a sense of balance. Any disturbance to the vestibular system could lead you to fall down, to be dizzy, or to have feelings of nausea and disorientation, as in car or motion sickness. This finely tuned system that adjusts your head and sense of uprightness by tuning into gravitational pulls is a kind of cosmic sense deep inside your skull.

You also have a *tactile* sense, which gives you information at the surface of your body. For example, you register hot or cold, hard or soft, rough or smooth, the irritation of an itch or the satisfaction of scratching, with your tactile sense.

You combine the information gathered by all these different types of senses to achieve complex actions. For example, if you play the piano, you must integrate your tactile feel for the keys with the teleceptor sense from your ears and with the proprioceptive sense of your muscles moving in your fingers and arms.

Since our culture, focused as it is on mirrors and photographs, is more oriented toward the teleceptors to provide feedback about the state of the body, you'll find this state of the body lesson quite different from what you may be used to, because you'll rely on all the internal senses to which you may not normally pay attention. The pressure of your body against the floor will serve the same function for your internal senses that a mirror serves for your visual sense of yourself through your eyes. This state of the body lesson allows you to capture extremely informative details about how you feel—more than your eyes can tell you about how you look. It takes a little practice, but you will notice things about yourself the first time you do this lesson that you probably have never been able to observe before and also could never see or hear or smell.

THE STATE OF THE BODY SCAN: THE FLOOR AS MIRROR

This body awareness exercise, practiced consistently, balances the body and releases tightness in all the major muscle groups. It is a wonderful starting point for making changes in your fitness, wellness, and vitality. Lying on the floor, you're able to observe the configuration and arrangement of your body in its most basic way—your posture when your body is most at rest. Imagine lying on firm, smooth sand. If you could be lifted from the sand and then could look down at the indentations you left in it, you would see a pattern in those indentations as unique as your signature. Most people don't realize that, even though they share features in common with many other people, their posture is completely unique. This "postural signature" is more than a physical signature: It is also a record of how your brain maps the muscular state of your body and maintains the habits of your posture.

Many people confuse position with posture. There is continuity in your posture no matter what position you are in. Your posture is an ongoing dynamic process that expresses itself in the way you stand, sit, or lie on the floor.

This is why people tend to have tension in the same muscle groups regardless of the position they're in. Your postural habits have been set into your bones, muscles, and brain and reproduce themselves regardless of your position, but there are distinct advantages to discovering your personal posture by lying on the floor.

When you lie on the floor, you get an opportunity to feel why certain parts of your body hold on and don't let go, even when you're lying down. Perhaps there are times when you think, "My neck keeps hurting on the right side," or, "My lower back pinches in a certain place all the time," and you don't really know why. Lying down permits you to reduce the muscle tone and to remove much of the customary strain and preoccupation of your nervous system as it organizes your standing and sitting postures.

Lying on the floor also helps counter some of the habitual stimulation that reinforces bad and ineffective muscular habits. Your body's unfelt twists, turns, and habits eventually present themselves in your regular activities, from cleaning the house to skiing, but it is hard to observe those movements when you are doing the activities.

Perhaps the most important advantage to lying on the floor is that the floor provides you with so many points of contact; it gives you the opportunity to feel much more of the network of your interconnected bones and muscles than you would be able to feel standing or sitting.

In a way you have probably never experienced, this exercise will help you get a sense of what areas of your body need attention and what age you feel you are. You will learn to observe the previously unobservable.

THE STATE OF THE BODY REPORT

Most people feel only a small amount of their posture. By practicing the State of the Body Scan, you will feel more of yourself. The lesson will also improve your posture and naturally relax your body. With more relaxed but greater attention over time, the Body Scan will improve your overall body awareness and lessen the slumping and scrunching that come from the habitual tensions that accelerate with aging.

Additionally, you will make your brain more flexible, which will help you to better retain what you learn and to maintain those changes for a longer period of time.

SOME THINGS TO REMEMBER

Read through the entire exercise first. You may want to record yourself reading the steps and then play the recording while you do the exercise.

Make sure you are wearing loose, comfortable clothing and are in a calm, quiet environment. Environment is key: When noise and distractions are at a minimum, you can enter into a quiet meditative state and observe distinctions in your body. Make sure you have a towel or a book handy so that your head can comfortably rest on the floor without straining your neck.

The scan can take as long as you like, but try to set aside at least 15 minutes so that you can really get into your observations.

You may find it useful to take notes on your observations, but don't get caught up in the details: It is more important to remember your sense of your body. Just as you don't record how you look after looking in the mirror, you don't need to record your observations as part of this scan.

I encourage you to use the floor as a kinesthetic mirror and to do a State of the Body Scan every day. In the same way that you look in the mirror to see what you look like, you can use the floor as a kinesthetic mirror to check in with how your body feels. You can use it during any of the movements described in Chapter 3 as a way of studying the effect of the program on your posture or just because it feels good, especially once you set yourself up comfortably.

1. Lie down on your back, with your arms down by your sides, your legs extended but relaxed, and your knees straight. Feel your contact with the floor. The aim is to lie in a position that is as close as possible to your natural standing position—a position that approximates how you would stand if you were about to walk somewhere. Keep your arms long and make sure both legs are extended. After all, when you are standing or walking, you usually don't keep your arms and legs crossed.

2. If this lying-down position is unfamiliar or uncomfortable for your back, modify it by bending your legs so that the bottoms of your feet are flat on the floor and you can balance your legs without leaning one against the other; your feet and ankles will be about a foot apart. If you find that your neck is strained, or if it feels too arched lying on your back, raise your head with a towel or book until you feel comfortable. A towel placed under a knee that feels strained when straight can also help, but first, lie down as instructed and check whether you need these supports. You don't want to cushion yourself to the point where you cannot feel your postural signature. Once you are comfortable, feel your contact against the floor with your arms, shoulders, back, buttocks, and feet.

3. Observe your postural signature—how your body rests on the floor in the posture you have while lying there.

   - Is there some part of your body that's pushing a little heavily into the floor?
   - Is there some part of your body that seems arched or high off the floor?
   - Notice the spaces between your body and the floor wherever they are, particularly those under your lower back and under your knees. Also notice where the floor supports you.
   - Are all of your muscles relaxed enough to allow as much support as possible from the floor?
   - As you scan the inside of your body and feel your contact with the floor, do some parts of yourself feel younger than other parts? You might find that the upper part of your body feels younger than your lower half. You might find that one leg or your head and neck have feelings that you unconsciously associate with feeling younger—for example, a feeling of dexterity or suppleness or agility. You would be a rare person if your whole body and all of its actions were aging evenly.
   - In this scan and throughout the program, you might find that the map of your body has many distinctions. Some parts of your body might feel twenty years younger than the rest of your body. It is

common to notice how your body feels older or looks older, but it can be more helpful to notice what's youthful about yourself. *By thinking of which parts of yourself feel most youthful, you orient your brain to be more youthful in all of your movements.*

4. Notice the "map" of the back surface of your body against the floor that is being made as you lie on the floor. For example, you might notice that there's more weight or a feeling of greater mass on one side of yourself compared to the other. You might feel that the left side is larger than the right, or vice versa. You might notice that your right leg feels heavier, thicker, or longer. However your right leg feels, compare it to the left leg. Which of your legs do you think would be easier to lift an inch off the floor? Which leg feels younger?

As you follow the program, you will find that your body's curvatures and sharp points of contact with the floor are changing. When your muscles are tight, your body curves more; this curvature decreases the points of contact between your body and the floor and makes each point carry more of the weight of your body. As your muscles relax, your body flattens itself more against the floor, creating more areas of contact, and the weight of your body is spread out.

At first, only 50 percent of the back surface of your body may actually be in contact with the floor if there is a large amount of space beneath the knees, the back, the neck, and the shoulders. As your muscles relax and get longer, these spaces shrink and a higher percentage of the back of your body will rest on the floor.

5. Notice how comfortable you are lying in this position. Are you at ease, or is your lower back hurting or starting to tighten? If you need to make your back more comfortable, remember that you can bend your knees and plant your feet on the floor with your legs far enough apart to be independently balanced.

6. Next, notice whether your neck is comfortable. Some people find that their neck is so arched that they're almost facing the wall behind them. This position of the neck may make breathing a little difficult. If this is the case, take a minute to place a small pillow, a couple of towels, or a book underneath your head. Find the amount of elevation that makes it a little easier to breathe and allows your neck to be more comfortable.

7. Return your attention to your body's pressure against the floor, which is also the floor's pressure against you. Observe which side of your body feels larger. If you were divided in half down your midline, is more of your body mass on the left side or the right side?

Then imagine that you are lying on a balance beam. If you fell asleep on this balance beam, which way would you roll off?

Which side of yourself feels younger? Why? What associations do you have with that side of your body?

As you imagine lying on the balance beam, you might feel that your pelvis is rolling or turning one way and your head and neck are going another. You might find your chest turning one way, as if on its own. These tendencies reveal your rotation habits—how you turn your body and orient your body when you're standing. These tendencies can be hard to feel when you're upright, and that is the advantage of the floor. This kinesthetic mirror reveals some things about your body and its organization that otherwise you might not notice.

8. Now let your mind focus on determining which are the areas of greatest contact between your body and the floor. The back of your rib cage? Your pelvis? Your head or your heels? When you put your attention on these contact points, your body will reduce the sharpness of those pressure areas and distribute your weight more evenly on the floor.

Just making this observation of your contact with the floor, of your back against the floor, leads your mind to reorganize the way you are holding your body on the floor and to spread your body's pressure from just a few areas to a more even distribution across your whole body. In other words, the awareness and observation of what you're doing actually creates a change—and you become more relaxed.

9. Put your attention on the places that are in contact with the floor but only a little bit, such as your heels or your calf muscles. As you observe these areas, notice whether one of your legs is straighter than the other one. You might find that the back of one knee is closer to the floor compared to the other one, or that one leg is turned open, meaning that it's rotated externally compared to the other one. One of your legs or a foot might be pointing straight up to the ceiling, which means that the muscles are working to hold the leg internally. You might be able to relate the sensation of your legs turning in or out to the sensation of which way your pelvis would roll if you were lying on a balance beam.

10. Finally, observe changes in the areas of pressure and your sense of position from the left to the right side of your body and note the percentage of your body that's resting on the floor. You don't need to move anything or adjust your body; just observe. This is a meditative and very practical way to relax.

The closer you get to the floor with your muscle tone, the more relaxed you are and the more your muscles unwind. If your muscles are wound up, they act like a bowstring. As you wind your muscles up (pulling back the bowstring), the bow of your body gets larger and your skeleton is higher off the floor. Unwinding your muscles allows your body to release into the floor.

You've now completed the State of the Body Scan. Take a few minutes to relax further and sit up when you are ready.

TOP VISIBLE SIGNS OF AGING

Our natural inclination is to look at wrinkles and sagging skin as the major visible signs of aging. However, the most difficult part of aging can be losing our freedom of movement and sinking into our most debilitating habits. These visible signs of aging appear as we start to lose the movement habits we learned as babies. Babies first learn the movement of front to back—for example, they see some food in front of them and bring it to their mouth. The next motor concept to develop is up-down movement as babies learn different ways to bring themselves to standing or sitting. Finally, infants learn lateral and spiral movements—how to turn, sidestep, or reach left or right.

As we age, we lose these motor concepts in the reverse order that we learned them as babies: First our lateral movement becomes more difficult or limited, then our ability to get up and down becomes compromised, and finally our movement options shrink to just dealing with what is in front of us. Happily, we can reverse this deterioration by unlearning some of our most unconscious movement habits and relearning more youthful and vital ways to move.

Here are some of the most common signs that reflect the loss of motor concepts. Check off the ones that apply to you and then take the following Change Your Age Mobility Survey, which explores how you live with these signs of aging in more detail.

_____ I have stiffness in my trunk and neck.

_____ I take more time and more steps to turn my whole body while walking.

_____ My lateral movement (being able to sway the pelvis or reach to either side) is lacking.

_____ I cannot lower myself safely and quickly to the floor and cannot rise quickly and effortlessly from the floor.

_____ I cannot rise quickly and effortlessly from a chair without pushing off with my hands.

_____ I have difficulty running across the street when I want.

_____ I have sore knees when climbing either up or down the stairs.

_____ I have a tendency to knock into things.

_____ I am no longer dancing or playing sports.

_____ I catch myself raising or hunching my shoulders.

_____ I feel awkward reaching up or bending down.

_____ My movements and breathing feel heavy.

_____ I feel hesitant or uncertain while initiating a movement.

CHANGE YOUR AGE MOBILITY SURVEY

These signs of aging can also be divided into several different categories of habits—postural habits, movement habits, timing habits, and balance habits. Understanding your habits can be the first step toward reversing the signs of aging and changing your age. The questions in the mobility survey will help you assess your functionality and gain insight into how aging manifests itself in your body. Take the survey, carefully considering each question and scoring accordingly. Mark your scores for each section and add up the total.

POSTURAL HABITS

1. Do you have difficulty turning your head to look from side to side?
Example: When you try to park your car, you can't look around easily to see what's behind you.

Never	Rarely	Sometimes	Often	Always
1	2	3	4	5

2. Do you have difficulty climbing up and down stairs?
Example: You have difficulty pushing through one leg to go up the stairs or it hurts your knee when you go down the stairs.

Never	Rarely	Sometimes	Often	Always
1	2	3	4	5

3. Do you have labored or shallow breathing?
Example: You notice, whether you're sitting or standing, that you occasionally take a sigh or deep breath. Sometimes you catch yourself holding your breath. People have told you that you're a shallow breather, and you seem to need these deep-breath breaks.

Never	Rarely	Sometimes	Often	Always
1	2	3	4	5

4. Do you have a protruding abdomen and an overly arched back?
Example: Sometimes you feel like you look fat, but you're not. You seem to be a fairly thin person with a big round stomach. Your lower back hurts when you stand.

Never	Rarely	Sometimes	Often	Always
1	2	3	4	5

5. Do you have a slumped posture?
Example: Sometimes, when you're sitting, you feel slumped in your chair. Occasionally you get pain in your neck just holding your head up. Sometimes when you're working at the computer your head is so far forward that your neck and shoulders start to get tight.

Never	Rarely	Sometimes	Often	Always
1	2	3	4	5

MOVEMENT HABITS

6. Do your movements feel heavy, as if someone turned up the gravity?
Example: You feel like you are moving through molasses. When you feel tense in your gut and tight in your back, you realize that you are lethargic. When you are more relaxed, you feel much lighter when you move.

Never	Rarely	Sometimes	Often	Always
1	2	3	4	5

7. Do you complain of having a stiff lower back and tight hips?
Example: Your back feels stiff and your hips don't swing, even if you dance or do other activities.

Never	Rarely	Sometimes	Often	Always
1	2	3	4	5

8. Do you get anxious about your balance when you reach up or look up?
Example: You can't seem to reach up to your higher kitchen cabinets any-more. When you use a step stool, you're worried that you might fall.

Never	Rarely	Sometimes	Often	Always
1	2	3	4	5

9. Do you find yourself pushing off with your hands to get out of a chair?
Example: You always get up by pushing with your hands into the armrests of your seat or sofa. It just seems natural—until you're in a situation where there are no arms to push off on. Then you have to use your legs, but you re-alize that your legs feel too weak or the movement is too uncomfortable.

Never	Rarely	Sometimes	Often	Always
1	2	3	4	5

10. Do you tend to stumble or shuffle when you walk?
Example: You shuffle instead of walk, hardly lifting your legs. You shuffle along so much that you often stub your toes.

Never	Rarely	Sometimes	Often	Always
1	2	3	4	5

TIMING HABITS

11. Do you have difficulty speeding up your movements?
Example: Sometimes you're concerned about crossing the street—worried that the light will change on you.

Never	Rarely	Sometimes	Often	Always
1	2	3	4	5

12. Do you find that your eyes move more slowly than they used to?
Example: It seems to take you a longer time to look around, as if you'll get dizzy if you move your eyes too fast. Or sometimes when you're walking through a mall you feel overstimulated, as though everything around you is moving too fast.

Never	Rarely	Sometimes	Often	Always
1	2	3	4	5

13. Do you have slower movements and a slower response time?
Example: You know you move more slowly than you used to, and you can't catch a fastball or return a serve as well as you once did.

Never	Rarely	Sometimes	Often	Always
1	2	3	4	5

BALANCE HABITS

14. Is it difficult for you to jump?
Example: You like to play basketball, but you don't land very well after a jump shot. Or perhaps even the thought of jumping seems impossible.

Never	Rarely	Sometimes	Often	Always
1	2	3	4	5

15. Is it difficult for you to hop on one leg?
Example: When you imagine hopping on one leg and turning in the air, it feels risky. If you are hiking, you feel uncomfortable hopping across a creek. Maybe you have hurt your knee while playing games with your kids.

Never	Rarely	Sometimes	Often	Always
1	2	3	4	5

16. Do you knock into things and even get bruises without knowing how?

Example: You often have bruises on your elbows and hands from walking into doorways or furniture, and you seem to sway from side to side when you walk. Or you notice that when you walk down a narrow hallway or airplane aisle, you sometimes veer left to right.

Never	Rarely	Sometimes	Often	Always
1	2	3	4	5

17. Is there a lack of sensation in your feet and legs, making you feel insecure about your balance?

Example: Sometimes you feel unsure of where your feet are; they just feel kind of fuzzy and like they're a long ways away. You find yourself looking down toward your feet when you walk.

Never	Rarely	Sometimes	Often	Always
1	2	3	4	5

18. Is it difficult for you to walk forward and backward so slowly that it takes 10 seconds to complete one step?

Example: You feel hesitant walking forward slowly and insecure walking backward. You might find it hard to move from one foot to the other very slowly because of difficulties balancing. Even following your partner's lead, dancing backward makes you feel uncertain.

Never	Rarely	Sometimes	Often	Always
1	2	3	4	5

Now tally your score. The lower your score, the greater your functional mobility is, while the higher your score, the more compromised your functional mobility is. If you score above 35, the Change Your Age Program will offer real benefits that can transform your life. Look at your scores for the different categories—postural habits, movement habits, timing habits, and balance habits—to get a sense of where you could focus your efforts.

Chapter 5 takes a closer look at these habits. Keep your scores handy: If your response to any of these questions was 3 or higher, consult Chapter 5 for tips on how to adjust your habits and for suggestions of particular lessons from Chapter 3 that will help you increase your mobility.

Retake this survey after completing Chapter 3. Then you will see how your score and your answers to the specific questions have changed, and you will also be able to make some concrete observations of changes in your body.

We have a more extensive version of this survey on our website (www.changeyourage.net), where these questions are placed in the context of a variety of movement activities. There you can also use your score to determine your Mobility Age and find more information on changing your age.

HOW OLD WOULD YOU LIKE TO BE?

Armed with the new internal sense of your body from the State of the Body Scan, the external assessment of your visible signs of aging, and a deeper understanding of your habits from the Change Your Age Mobility Survey, try this Change Your Age thought exercise: How old would you like to be? People who have completed this program find that not only can they reclaim abilities and agilities they thought they lost years ago, but they can also move more smoothly, more fluidly, and more gracefully than they ever have before.

I remember a 50-year-old man with knee and back problems who had given up skiing and golfing. Or the 60-year-old San Francisco woman dealing with the very practical issues that arose from living at the top of a hill and not being sure her weak ankles would hold up so that she could stay in her home. And I remember the basically fit couple who continued going to the gym together several times a week but were feeling stiffer and older despite all their exercise.

All of these people learned to move more easily by first believing that they could change their functional age and then setting realistic goals. All of them began to move and to live like they had done years earlier. The 50-year-old man with knee and back problems has gone back to skiing and golfing. The San Francisco hill-dweller now goes on hikes and finds the hills of San Francisco energizing. The basically fit couple has found through the Change Your Age Program that they both move as though they were 10 to 15 years younger.

However you see your current fitness and health, before you begin, it's important to really think about what it would mean to you to "change your age." Remember, you probably won't move like a teenager again, but almost anyone can move better than they did five years ago and learn to move more gracefully than they ever have before.

- What is your dream for a younger self?
- What would you like to do better?
- How would you like to feel?
- How specific can you make this dream of a younger self?
- How would you know if you had achieved this dream?

Perhaps you would like to have less pain. So ask yourself: How much less pain? What would be a marker? Then ask yourself: How much younger would it make me feel if I were successful?

It's amazing how extremely specific people can get about what this idea means to them. One woman in a workshop wanted to experience less lower back pain. She narrowed her goal down to being able to stand on her feet for an hour without pain. She felt that this would take 15 years off her age.

Another woman wanted to be able to run for an hour at a time. It was her dream of youth. For her, that would take 12 years off her age.

A man with intermittent and cyclical problems with his knees and a nagging foot injury didn't mind giving up long runs, but he wanted to know that he could do his basic exercise routine, including long walks and short jogs, whenever he felt like it. He felt that this would take 8 years off his age.

These are the sort of concrete, realistic dreams of a younger self that I am talking about. I can't overstate the importance of *thinking* about your body and your age. It is your brain that tells you how you feel and how you experience your life. If you ignore your body and accept your aches, pains, and stiffness as unchangeable signs of aging, your beliefs will continue to limit what you do, how you feel, and how you think. As you begin to think about your body and physical health, you can begin to take control and live the life you want. If you know that you can simply and easily feel 5, 10, or 15 years younger, you have all the motivation you need to begin to change your age.

Now that you have learned some tools to gain a greater understanding of your body and set some goals for how you want to change your age, let's begin the Change Your Age Program.

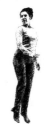

CHAPTER THREE

THE CHANGE YOUR AGE PROGRAM

The Everyday Ultimate Body-Brain Conditioning Program—
30 Basic Exercises

THERE ARE five core positions in the program—lying down, sitting, kneeling, crouching, and standing. In this chapter, you will find detailed instructions for all five positions. Advanced variations are offered for some of these lessons, but don't feel pressured to do them before you are ready. You will be able to measure your rejuvenation by your ability to expand the variety of movements you can perform with comfort and ease.

These lessons can be performed every day, although it would take a long time to do all 30 of them. As you are learning them, don't bite off more than you can chew. Performing a few lessons a day and returning the next day to do more is the best approach to learning for your brain and body. You want to finish learning the lessons feeling good when you then return to your State of the Body Scan from Chapter 2. In Chapter 4, you will find targeted lesson sequences that you can do each day after you've learned the Change Your Age Program.

Before you start a lesson, read through it and look to the photos for guidance. This mental rehearsal will help you unleash your physical imagination. You might discover that where you have difficulty visualizing a movement, you also have difficulty performing that movement; by taking time to imagine the movement, you will actually help yourself when it is time to move your body. Recent research has proven that clearly imagining a movement without actually moving stimulates and grows neurons, enabling you to improve your movement more than if you spent an equal amount of time physically practicing it.

You can even do most of the program with your eyes closed, which might make it easier for you to visualize the movements. When we close our eyes, we heighten our kinesthetic and tactile senses. Of course, it would be difficult to read this book with your eyes closed, so you could record yourself reading a lesson and listen to the recording as you perform the movement.

I also encourage you to work with a partner or a small group of friends, reading the lessons to each other. This can be a lot of fun for many people because you learn by watching other people move and discussing what you experienced.

This program asks you to be intuitive and instinctual and to trust yourself. Unlike other fitness books, you won't find strict rules on repetitions or time limits here; I'll suggest parameters, but this program is about being in touch with your body and brain—and your sense of movement. If you devote time to counting repetitions or try to complete a lesson within a certain time frame, you will deny your brain the opportunity to experience the subtle changes that are taking place in yourself. Counting distracts us from sensing.

HOW TO PREPARE FOR A LESSON

Before you begin, here are a few important tips for getting the most out of the lessons:

GO SLOWLY

Take your time—you'll learn more! These movements may seem unusual and unfamiliar. You will need time to assimilate them and to feel the way your body is moving and changing. Do not rush! Pause whenever you feel like it, and repeat movements you find pleasurable or want to experience more fully.

INSIST ON COMFORT

There is no reward in doing any of the movements in an uncomfortable position. Gently alter your position in whatever way makes it comfortable for you. I want you to enjoy the process of the movement as much as the result. If it hurts, it's not helping you. Never try to override pain if you feel it. Pain is your body's way of asking you to find a new way to move. Answer it with gentleness and respect.

DON'T COMPETE WITH YOURSELF

The Change Your Age Program is not about seeing how far you can move, how high you can lift, or how long you can stretch. Your goal should be to discover *how* your body achieves a movement so that you can learn to make that movement easier. Your movements should always be as light and effortless as possible. Imagine how good it will feel to do simple mobile tasks without stress and strain.

USE YOUR IMAGINATION

Allow the movement to become very clear and lucid in your mind, like a scene from a movie. You may find that your body responds to your mind by moving as if it is replaying the imagined movement, with almost no effort at all.

REST FREQUENTLY

These movements, while gentle and pleasurable, may cause slight strain because you are using parts of muscles you may not have used in a long time, or you may be using them in ways that are not familiar. Rest often during each lesson. You cannot rest too much. Resting is a time when your brain can integrate new movements and new sensations. Relax and let the movement settle in. Enjoy the feeling. Who knows—it could become a habit.

CHOOSE A COMFORTABLE SPACE

Learning occurs in direct proportion to the comfort and relaxation your body experiences during the movements. In other words, if you feel comfortable from the beginning of a new lesson, you are much more likely to learn it. For this reason, it is perfectly all right for you to do lying-down lessons in bed if you find the floor uncomfortable or if getting up and down from the floor causes stress or pain.

If you are doing the lessons on the floor, please use an exercise mat or carpeted floor rather than a hard floor, and have available a towel you can use as a neck or knee support if needed. Make sure that you have space around you to move and that your clothes are loose enough to not restrain your movement. It is important to lower the lights and decrease distracting outside noises so you can sense the reactions and changes your body will experience.

DON'T FEEL OBLIGATED TO DO ALL OF THE LESSONS

Some lessons may be difficult or painful for you to perform, either from the starting position or at some point during the lesson. If you feel discomfort or pain while moving, stop. Just imagining doing the lesson, or parts of the lesson, will benefit you almost as much as physically performing the movements. Then, as your body changes and your quality of motion improves, go back to the tricky lesson to see whether it has now become possible to perform it in some way. If the movements still cause pain, stop and choose a lesson that does not.

TAKE THE LESSONS WITH YOU

Pay close attention to how each lesson affects you throughout your day. Notice changes in the way you reach, walk, sit, and think. A lesson doesn't have to end with its last movement—let the learning process linger and grow. I strongly advise keeping a journal to note the changes you observe after each lesson. You might want to repeat a lesson that gave you a particularly interesting or pleasurable feeling.

POSITION 1: LYING DOWN

Most of your youngest movements were done lying down. You probably don't remember when you learned to roll on your back, to roll from side to side, or to lie on your back and turn your head to look all around the room. Then there was that time when you rolled over all the way to your stomach. Incredible! Only to discover that, with some exploration and practice, you could roll all the way onto your back again. Wow—a much bigger world.

Back in those days you learned not only how to bring your hands to your mouth and other neat tricks but how to push against the floor, at first with your arms and then later with your feet, back, belly, and bottom.

In these lessons, you will return to the days of your early movements.

POSITION 1: LYING DOWN ON YOUR BACK

The program begins with lying down on your back to ground yourself. "Grounding" refers to a general feeling of stability, a connection to the earth, a certain kind of awareness. It also refers to gravity and, as I teach it, to "ground forces," which are the forces you press against the ground in order to move your body. (For example, you must push down to jump up; you must pull backward to step forward.) Most of your ability to propel yourself through the world starts belly down, a position that allows you to push with your arms and legs.

You can see the power of ground forces at work when you watch astronauts struggling to move deliberately in zero gravity, or when you watch divers pushing against the platform to perform their amazing moves. Without ground forces, movement is difficult.

Lesson 1: COORDINATING YOUR NECK AND EYES WITH YOUR LEGS AND PELVIS

● **Intention:** To differentiate (discriminate) the motion of your eyes from the motion of your head, neck, shoulders, and pelvis. This lesson will help you if you can't move your eyes or turn your head easily and quickly, which is one of the first obvious signs of aging.

● **Starting Position:** Lie on your back with your arms on the floor at the level of your shoulders and your legs long. I recommend closing your eyes so that you can go further into your kinesthetic sense. Your eyes and your visual sense can often pull you out and make it more difficult to sense your body.

1. Roll your head a little bit from side to side, searching for the ease in the movement.

   Most of the time when we turn our heads from side to side, we turn as far as we can turn. Here, rather than think about which side allows you to turn your head farther, find the side on which it is simply easier to turn. When you discover that easier side, the side that feels more natural, roll your head back to the center.

Change Your Age Tip: To detect a lightness, an easiness in movement, we have to reduce the effort in our muscular contractions. The harder we try to do something, the more difficult it becomes to make distinctions. While you're working to feel which is the lighter side, can you make that side even easier and lighter?

   Roll your head only to the side that is easier. Do so a few times until the movement becomes even easier and smoother.

   Rest your head wherever it feels most comfortable.

   So, did you find the side you prefer? Recognizing which side is easier helps you to understand some of your established habits.

2. Still lying down, pull your left leg up toward the ceiling so that you are "standing" on your left foot with your left knee bent. Can you push through your left foot to lift the left side of your pelvis and roll it to the right? You can shift the placement of your foot to find the easiest place to roll your pelvis. Your head may roll to the right, or it may feel easier rolling to the left. Go with whatever feels natural to you as long as you are aware of how you are moving.

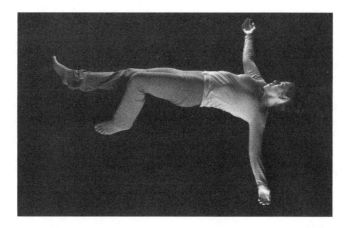

Make it an easy push. Feel how pushing through that foot carries a twist up through your body that may facilitate the rolling of your head. Allow your head to roll farther.

Discover how the use of your legs and pelvis helps your head to turn more easily.

3. Rest with your arms and legs long. Roll your head from side to side again. Notice if your sense of the movement of your head and neck has expanded. Maybe rolling your head has gotten easier on both sides?

Change Your Age Tip: Differentiation is a brain-body concept that everybody uses and everybody needs.

For example, to type or play the piano, you must learn to differentiate the movements of your fingers from each other in specific ways. If you didn't, your hands would move as if you were wearing a mitten.

When you turn your head to look at something, your eyes can move only a certain amount inside your head, and then your head begins to turn. If you want to see still farther in back of yourself, you need to turn your trunk and move your shoulders, and if you're standing, you'll probably need to shift your weight.

Most people have been taught to think of stretching their muscles to increase their range and ease of movement, but stretching muscles will not help you improve a skill, especially if that skill involves sitting more easily, climbing stairs more lightly, or walking more gracefully. For example, if you want to speak more clearly or learn to sing, it would be absolutely useless to grab hold of your tongue and stretch it by pulling it out of your mouth.

The more differentiated your neck becomes through proper use, along with your eyes, shoulders, and trunk, the farther you'll be able to turn as you involve more components or parts of your body in the same movement.

---

4. Return to the same arrangement (lying on the floor, left knee bent so that you are standing on your left foot and your arms are out to your sides). This time open your eyes and look with a soft focus toward the ceiling. Push through your left foot and let your head roll as before, to either side, but keep your eyes oriented toward the ceiling. Your head may go so far that eventually it gets hard to see exactly where you started.

   Feel that your foot is solidly in contact with the floor. Feel that you can know how you are positioning and moving your legs, your pelvis, and your shoulders. Think about whether your arms are too close to the sides of your body.

   Now perform the whole sequence of pushing through your foot and rolling your pelvis and head a little faster.

   Do your eyes have the independence to soft-focus on the ceiling while your head is rolling on the floor? Your eyes can work independently from the muscles of your neck and trunk. Some people can turn their head to one side, and their shoulders, pelvis, and the leg they are standing on will follow. For other people, their body will follow the movement of their eyes. Part of what you are learning is to create more independence between your feet, trunk, head, neck, shoulders, and eyes.

   Come to rest with your arms and legs down. While resting, observe the differences in your impression on the floor, as you did in the State of the Body Scan. Does one leg feel younger than the other? Do you feel that your body is inclined to roll more easily toward one side? Maybe one leg feels longer. Slowly roll your head from side to side with your eyes closed and feel whether you favor one side.

   Slowly come to standing. Observe the differences in standing and walking between the two sides of your body. Which leg feels younger? Does your head turn more easily to one side?

Go back to the floor and again lie with your arms out to the side and your legs long.

5. Now bend your right knee and stand on your right foot. Let your eyes close, if you want. Can you find an easy way to push your right foot into the floor and feel how your pelvis starts to roll to the left and then how your head eventually rolls?

Feel the influence of your rolling pelvis on the movement of your head. You might discover that your head can roll more easily in either direction.

And then pause for a few seconds.

Can you open your eyes? While your eyes are looking up above your-self, continue the same movement of rolling your pelvis and your head.

Don't worry about rolling your head farther. Instead, observe that your head can roll and your eyes can stay looking at the ceiling. Try to make it easy. You want to make sure that you are able to maintain the position of your eyes, keeping them focused on the ceiling, even as you turn your head.

Pause. Take a full rest for 30 seconds or a minute, with your arms and legs long.

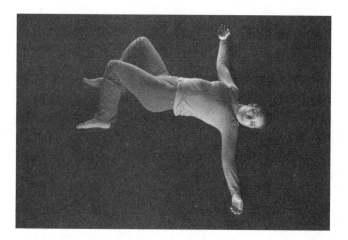

6. Now bend both knees and "stand" both feet on the floor. Keep your feet a comfortable distance apart so that your legs are independently balanced above them.

Next, can you tilt your knees over toward the right side? As you do this, your feet will keep some contact with the floor. Your pelvis will roll as your knees tilt. Then, return your knees to the upright position and repeat the movement. Keep breathing and observe whether you can relax your jaw.

Pause, with your feet still in standing position.

7. Repeat Step 6 on the left side. On which of the two sides is it easier to do this movement? Explore this a few times until you feel the difference.

8. Now, with both feet "standing," slowly tilt your knees from side to side and notice that your head is inclined to roll. Maybe your head wants to stay in the middle, or wants to follow the direction of your knees, or wants to go the opposite way. Any of these inclinations is fine. What is most important is that you are observing what you are doing.

When you keep your eyes softly focused above yourself while tilting your legs from side to side, you'll continue to differentiate the muscles in your eyes, neck, and back. Don't let your eyes freeze the motion of your pelvis. Let your eyes, calm and still, be a part of the movement, just as the rest of your body can be calm and in motion. Make sure you keep breathing while you do this, so as to gain mobility in your ribs.

9. Rest with your arms and legs long.

Tune in to your contact with the floor and to the general state of your body. Notice whether your body feels younger. Do parts of you feel younger than other parts? Turn your head slowly from side to side and see whether this movement is any easier.

Rest. When you are ready, come to a full stand.

Stand easily and look around the room. Do you feel as if your visual field has expanded? As you walk, see whether you feel a difference in your balance as you walk turning your head from side to side. After doing this lesson, maybe you would feel safer crossing the street in heavy traffic or hiking on a rocky trail.

This might be a good time to journal, draw, or, if you are with a friend, discuss what you learned and experienced in this lesson.

Lesson 2: RELEASING THE HIPS INTO PLEASURE

● **Intention:** To find a comfortable and pleasurable way of releasing excess work in the stiff muscles of your inner legs and hips.

● **Starting Position:** Lie on your back with your arms down at your sides and your legs long.

1. Feel the pressure under your heels and notice whether you feel more pressure from the floor touching your left heel compared to your right. Is the pressure on the outside of the heel more apparent on one side than the other? Also observe the pressure under your calf muscles. Does that pressure help tell you which of your two legs is pointed more to the ceiling and which is pointed more to the outside? Make sure your legs are relaxed. Don't try to hold them in any particular way.

2. Very gently turn your right leg farther to the right and let your knee softly bend so that the outside edge of your right foot begins to slide on the floor up toward you. Then slide the edge of your foot back down the same track it went up. Repeat the movement several times, very slowly, searching for the path of least resistance and effort as you slide the outside edge of your foot up and down on the floor.

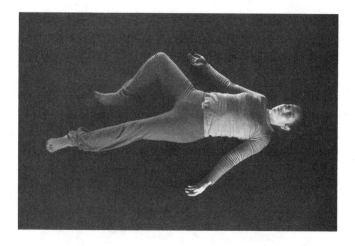

Change Your Age Tip: As you slide your foot up and down, make sure your knee hangs open completely so that there's no work happening in the inner muscles of your thigh. The more unnecessary muscular work you perform, the more difficult, heavy, and resistant the movement of the leg becomes. Every so often let your leg rest, with your knee bent and your foot pulled up, to make sure you are letting go of your inner thigh muscles.

After exploring the movement of sliding the edge of your right foot up and down the floor, rest and observe what has changed in the way your leg rests on the floor. Is your leg softer? Is it pointing in a different direction than earlier? Does your hip feel softer? You might even find that your lower back has released to the floor on the right side.

3. Perform the same exploration of this soft and lazy movement on the left side. Is it easier or harder than on the right? Notice whether your eyes or even your head want to move to the left when you move your left leg up and down. Rest. Feel the expansion in your pelvis and the release of excess work in your legs. Pause with your legs long and arms down at your sides.

4. Turn both of your legs open, with the knees hanging apart, and slide the outside edges of both of your feet up toward yourself at the same time. As you go up and down this way, slowly and gently, feel what your back and your pelvis are doing to assist the movement.

As the edges of your feet slide up, keep some distance between them.

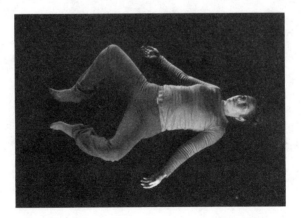

5. Rest with your arms on the floor above your head and your elbows slightly bent out to the sides. Once again, slide the outside edges of both feet up toward yourself and leave them there with your knees hanging open. Now let your head easily roll from side to side while breathing deeply.

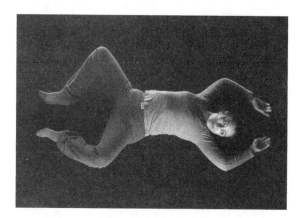

Rest in this position, with the knees suspended and the arms open, and feel the comfort of being like a baby sleeping on the floor. Let your ribs move freely as you breathe. If letting your knees hang open feels uncomfortable, place a pillow under the side of each knee to give yourself more support.

Lesson 3: USING YOUR ABDOMEN TO RELEASE YOUR BACK

● **Intention:** To gain greater flexibility and maximum length in your back. Before you start, do the State of the Body Scan and feel your contact with the floor. Notice the curves in your spine, the parts of your body that touch the floor, and the parts that don't. Remember this feeling because it might change significantly after this lesson.

When we do abdominal exercises like sit-ups, only the strongest part of our abdominal muscle fibers gets stronger, while the weaker parts become relatively weaker. This lesson strives to engage all parts of the abdomen.

● **Starting Position:** Lie on your back with your arms down at your sides, both knees bent and both feet standing on the floor. Feel that your legs can be independently balanced so that your ankles and knees are as wide apart as your hips.

1. Gently lift your head to look toward your feet. Notice the amount of effort it takes to perform this movement. Don't strain by holding the position. Put your head down again. Lift your head another time or two, only to notice how much effort is involved and how high your head can go without struggling.

2. Completely interlace the fingers of your hands and place them behind your head. Feel that you are supporting your head and part of your neck. Lift your head while aiming your elbows toward your knees. Do this gently and easily without straining your abdominal muscles. Then set your head back down and let your elbows return to the floor. This movement is not like a sit-up or an abdominal crunch.

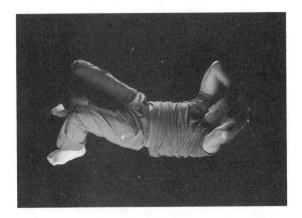

Change Your Age Tip: If you find that your neck is strained from pulling on your head too hard, move your hands farther down toward your neck so that the neck itself is supported throughout the movement.

3. Keeping your fingers interlaced and your elbows away from the floor, again lift your head several times and look at your knees as you use your arms and head together. Feel what happens to your back and

pelvis. Do they move? Feel your abdominal muscles contracting, very softly. Can you feel your back rocking on the floor?

Rest with your arms and legs long.

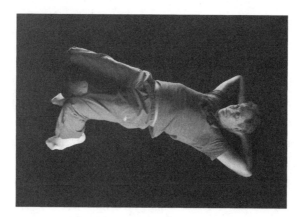

4. Return your feet to the standing position and again interlace your fingers behind your head with your elbows apart. Push with your feet into the floor so that you can slowly and easily lift your pelvis from the floor. Do this several times, somewhere between five and ten times, but don't get caught up in counting off repetitions. As always, the most important thing is to feel, to be aware of your body.

There is no need to lift the pelvis as high as you possibly can; the idea is to lift your pelvis as high as it takes to feel weight on your upper back. Can you feel the muscles of your buttocks working?

Pause with your pelvis resting on the floor.

5. Now lift your head again to point your elbows to your knees and simultaneously lift your pelvis in the air. Eventually, if you lift your pelvis high enough, you will feel your head needing to lower to the floor. At that point, lift your head until you feel your pelvis needing to lower to the floor. It becomes a seesawlike movement. Practice this movement several times.

As you do this movement, maintain a constant distance between your pelvis and your head. When your head rises a bit, your pelvis naturally lowers a bit, and vice versa. Don't lower your pelvis until you feel you have to, and don't lower your head until you feel you have to. You will be rocking along the entire length of your spine, and every section of your abdominal muscles will have a chance to wake up.

Rest for a while on your back with your arms and legs long. Take time to feel the contact between your back and the floor.

● *Body Intelligence Reminder for Advanced Variation on Lesson 3:*
● You may find some of the variations and some of the lessons difficult
● because you haven't yet learned the body awareness to perform them well. Practice these lessons slowly, making sure you don't force yourself to achieve something for which you haven't established a feeling or a felt sense. Don't compete with yourself.

Perform these movements only a few times. There is no advantage to doing many repetitions of the same movements. Many people find that they can feel more after four or five repetitions of a movement. If you do the same movement too much and for too long, however, your attention is likely to wander and your awareness will go out the window.

By practicing some of the lessons you find more difficult, you will increase your body awareness and these lessons will become easy.

Advanced Variation on Lesson 3:
USING YOUR ABDOMEN TO RELEASE YOUR BACK

● **Intention:** To create maximum strength in your core abdominal muscles and release the back from any habitual stiffness.

● **Starting Position:** Lie on your back, leaving your pelvis on the floor. Bring your knees above yourself. Interlace your fingers again and put them behind your neck.

1. Slowly draw your elbows and knees toward each other. Some people are able to touch their elbows to their knees. If you're touching, remain with your elbows touching your knees. If you're very flexible, you might be able to grasp the outside of your knees with your elbows.

Otherwise, and for most people, find a comfortable relationship between your elbows and knees and then imagine that you are supporting a stick between each elbow and knee.

2. Without changing the configuration you're in, can you very slowly roll a small distance from side to side? Go as long as you want, but make sure you can still breathe easily!

3. Rest on your back with your arms and legs long. Feel how your body contacts the floor now compared to the beginning of the lesson.

Lesson 4: SEESAW BREATHING

● **Intention:** To recognize the movements of your ribs, your diaphragm, your abdomen, the sides of your body, and even your back—all the parts of yourself that move when you breathe. Most people tend to move quite a lot in certain parts of their torso as they breathe, while other parts don't move at all. In this lesson, you will learn to involve more parts of yourself in your breathing motion.

● **Starting Position:** Lie on your back, stretch out your legs, and put your arms down at your sides. Put a pillow or towel underneath your head, or under both your head and neck, to make yourself as comfortable as possible.

1. Observe the movement of your breathing without changing anything. As soon as we begin to watch our breathing, we tend to alter it, so don't inhale more or faster than usual.

    What parts of your torso expand the most? What parts don't seem to be involved? If I told you that I don't believe you ever breathe, how would you prove to me that you do? How do you know you're breathing? Do you identify with the feeling of air passing through your nostrils and going down your throat?

2. Fill your lungs with air as much as you comfortably can. Breathe fully in and out this way and observe what happens to your lower back. As you inhale, do you feel any tendency for the hollow of your back to rise from the floor? As you breathe out, does your lower back go down toward the floor? Do you feel your waistline moving out to the sides?

Or does your torso seem to move toward the ceiling without any tendency to expand backward or to the sides?

Change Your Age Tip: Instead of increasing the actual volume of the chest in accordance with its structure, many people raise their chest by raising their lower back from the floor. Inhaling this way does not allow the breastbone—or sternum—to move relative to the spine. As you observe yourself breathing, don't change anything. The goal here is not to impose a particular idea of breathing on you, but to help you become aware of how you move so that you can learn to make adjustments that are more organic and go far deeper.

---

3. Bend your knees and stand your feet on the floor, near yourself, with the feet apart and each leg independently balanced. Place one hand on your belly and the other hand on your chest, keeping your elbows on the floor. Take a comfortable full breath of air and hold it. Without letting any air in or out, push that air down as though you were sending it out between your legs. Feel how your belly and waist expand. Still without breathing, pull your belly in and let your chest expand again. Go back and forth like this, slowly pushing the air down toward the bottom of your pelvis, and then up toward the top of your chest.

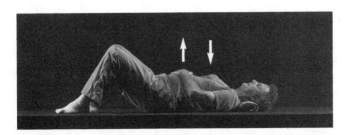

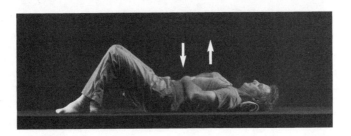

Go back and forth slowly, gently, and steadily. You might discover that your hands go up and down, alternating like a seesaw. Breathe whenever you need to. Please don't challenge yourself to see how long you can hold your breath.

When you need to breathe, simply break the cycle completely and rest for a while. Don't try to do more than five or six movements back and forth before you stop and rest.

Change Your Age Tip: Holding your breath and pushing the air up and down requires the participation of all the muscles of the ribs, shoulders, chest, back, belly, and pelvis.

In this lesson, you'll transform your old breathing habits by using more muscles than people ordinarily use when they breathe, muscles that should be involved in breathing. When you've learned this lesson, you'll find that more of your body participates in your breathing. In a sense, you'll be waking up your torso to its full potential for moving with your breath.

---

4. Roll onto your hands and knees and come to a crawling position. Keeping your hands where they are on the floor, lower your pelvis toward your heels, with your chest facing the floor and your legs. You can rest your head on the floor and part of your chest on or between your thighs. In this position, notice your breathing and lower back. Your back may now feel as though it's lifting to the ceiling and out to the sides. As you take deep breaths in this position, you might even feel your back expanding all the way down to your hips. Remain in this position for at least 10 seconds, just long enough to observe your breathing.

   Leave this position and return to resting on your back.

5. Once again bend your knees and balance them above your feet. Put your hands on your waistline so that your thumbs are pointing toward your back and your fingers are around your waist toward the front. Breathe in again and hold the breath. Pass the air down to your pelvis. Does it feel like you are pushing out in all directions with your belly, not just to the ceiling?

   Can you feel the distance between your fingers and thumbs widen as you push? Now pull your belly in to expand your chest. Can you feel your thumbs and fingers coming together? Pass the air back and forth through your torso several times while observing how your back reaches to the floor, as well as how the air travels both forward and to the sides of your torso. Remember not to challenge yourself to hold your breath any longer than is comfortable.

You can also practice Step 5 of this movement while sitting or standing, thus reinforcing good breathing habits in all positions.

End this lesson by breathing normally for a while. It's all right if "breathing normally" seems rather confusing right now. Your breathing will be altered by this lesson. Observe how it's different from before.

POSITION 1: LYING DOWN ON YOUR STOMACH

Most of us prefer to do exercises while lying on our back and find it a strange feeling to lie on our stomach. But this position develops core strength. Having the floor beneath us gives us something to push off from, and there are many exercises that are extremely beneficial done from this position. Think of all the push-ups that babies do before they learn how to sit up!

In order to win in judo, for instance, you want to get your opponent onto his back because we lose our strength—our "power"—in that position. In this program, you'll practice not only by lying on your stomach but also by moving from side to side, waking your body up with new movements. You will feel a renewed sense of strength and flexibility, and the results will be apparent in a body that feels highly energized.

Lesson 5: ROLLING INTO LENGTH
ACROSS YOUR STOMACH

● **Intention:** To learn how to get comfortable on your stomach and how to move easily off your stomach if you feel uncomfortable. This lesson is most easily done on a relatively friction-free surface. Many people are told not to lie on their stomach. This may temporarily be a good idea for those who have recently undergone some kinds of surgeries or suffered certain injuries, but it's not a position to avoid completely for the rest of your life.

● **Starting Position:** Lie on your right side with your knees and hips bent.

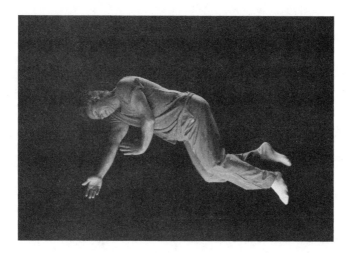

1. Place your left hand on the floor and put your left foot on the floor in front of your right foot, keeping your knees stacked on top of each other.

   Slide your feet away from yourself, with the intention of straightening both legs, and slide your left hand along the floor up above your head as you slowly roll onto your stomach. Control the roll so that you don't flop onto your stomach. Feel that you can leverage yourself at any point. Return to the starting position of lying on your side.

   Repeat the beginning of this movement, but before rolling all the way onto your stomach, practice sliding your hands and feet toward each other so that you return to your right side.

   Practice going back and forth toward your stomach and back to your side a few times, without going all the way onto your stomach. Search for the feeling of control and reversibility—for the way you would organize yourself to prevent yourself from rolling down a hill too fast.

A PRINCIPLE OF MOVEMENT

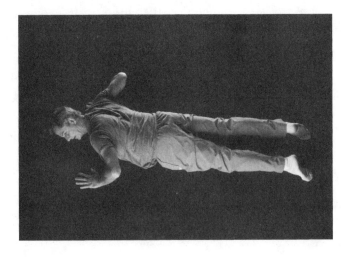

Acontrolled movement is reversible: You can return with complete control through the trajectory that your body has made. For example, in this lesson, if many photographs were taken of you rolling onto your stomach and returning to your side, the viewer would not be able to distinguish which direction you were going because your movement, if controlled, would be completely reversible.

A movement that is not reversible is one that involves momentum or rapid acceleration, such as throwing a ball. Catching a ball is not the reverse of throwing a ball.

• • •

Rest on your stomach for a little while with your arms above your head and your legs long. Put your head and arms in any position that makes you feel comfortable.

Observe how you breathe on your stomach. Breathing is a critical thing to do immediately after rolling onto your stomach, especially if you are not used to being in that position. Feel the ease of breathing on your stomach. Notice how your back expands.

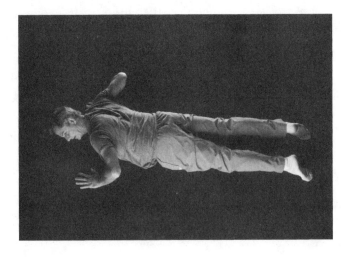

2. In a motion just long enough to enable you to take a breath, and with your hands in a push-up position, lift your head, look in front of yourself, turn your head to one side, and rest on your cheek for a moment.

   Turn your head to the other side. Practice resting your head comfortably on the floor on either cheek.

3. Roll onto your right side again, sweeping your arms and your feet toward each other. Repeat the movement of sliding your hands and feet apart, rolling onto your stomach, and returning to your side as often as you would like.

   If the movement feels effortful, as if the floor is providing too much friction, play with continuously integrating the actions of your pelvis, arms and hands, and legs and feet. Your brain may organize the movement more efficiently if you use the image of folding and unfolding your body. You may have to emphasize some parts of your body at a slightly different time than is spontaneous at first. Eventually, the movement should feel like a very light and easy way to roll onto your side and return to your stomach, but it does require deepening your sensations and using your fullest attention and awareness.

THE IMPORTANCE OF ORIENTATION AND SCANNING

Any living being that needs to locate food, water, temperature differences, fresh air, its own nest, or other nests needs to have a sense of orientation. Without a strong sense of orientation, all animal life would have a difficult time moving around because no creatures would know where to go. This affects all human movement as well. People need to turn left and right to scan or search the environment around themselves. What we think of as coordinated movement means that all the parts are moving together in a cooperative manner. But what are the parts cooperating for?

In upright posture, humans must have the left-and-right scanning movement readily available so that they can locate anything of importance or interest in the environment by quickly and easily turning the head: "Mmmm, smells good, let's go that way"; or "Look, food in that direction"; or "Did you hear that? I think it's coming from our left—let's look." Foundational to our ability to see, hear, and smell is an orientational turning of the neck, whether toward something pleasant or away from possible danger.

Your brain and your senses start most of the movements of your body. For example, turning your head left and right is built into the anatomy of your neck and the placement of your eyes and ears and, of course, your mouth and nose.

When you scan the environment with difficulty because your neck is stiff or tight or your eyes move sluggishly, you cannot scan the environment effectively. When taking the safety measure of searching for traffic before crossing a street, many people first scan the street and then walk across without turning their head. Walking, which involves balancing, is simply too hard for most people—even very young people—to do while simultaneously turning the head and scanning the environment. Almost anyone can learn to walk at a pace independent from the speed with which they might turn their head.

Here is a simple test: Walk and turn your head from side to side, even in your own house, and you'll find that your head speed tends to match your stepping speed; whichever is slower becomes dominant. If you walk fast, your head moves more slowly relative to your feet.

An important goal of these movement lessons is to help you make the turning motions of your head completely independent from your stepping.

● ● ●

Lesson 6: REGAINING FULL USE OF YOUR NECK

● **Intention:** To turn your head fully and painlessly. Practicing this lesson for only a few minutes a week will restore and maintain the kind of neck rotation you may have had only when you were very young.

This particular movement is very useful if you can't turn or bend your head or neck easily. Neck rotation is often a little more limited lying on your back, but more motion can be obtained while lying on your stomach. Like all animals, you will find that complex orienting responses are most easily and naturally developed while lying on the belly.

● **Starting Position:** Lie on your back.

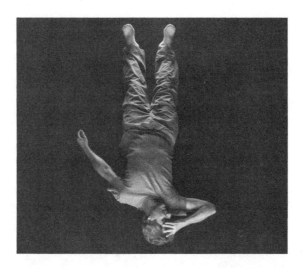

1. Put the palm of your right hand on your forehead with your elbow pointing out to the side. Imagine that you have a board from your fingertips to your elbow and that your head is a cylinder or a ball. Now, can you roll your head underneath your hand by pushing with your arm and hand? As you roll your head to the left, you should be pushing down toward the wrist end of your hand, and as you pull your head back in the other direction, you should roll toward your fingertips.

   Make sure that your head feels completely passive, that your neck is doing no activity or work, and that all the work is being done by the power of your arm. You should feel the skin on your forehead sliding across the bone of your skull before you feel any movement of your head. If you feel the skin pulled to the limit across the bone and then finally your head beginning to move, you'll know that your arm is doing the work. Let your jaw relax and your eyes go soft. Now set your arm down. Leave it and rest.

2. Put your left hand on your forehead and point your elbow to the left. Move your head with your left hand in the same way as you did with your right. See that you minimize the work in your neck. If you can learn not to compress the joints by overcontracting the neck muscles, then you can gain mobility and freedom.

    Leave the movement and let your arm rest at your side. Do you notice any difference in the quality or condition of your neck?

3. Now roll over onto your stomach and put your forehead on the floor, with your hands in push-up position. Your hands will be a little wider than your shoulders, and your elbows will be pointing toward the ceiling, as though you were going to push up. See that your feet are apart.

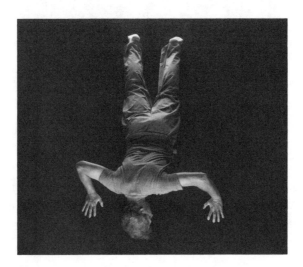

4. Slowly roll across your forehead and onto your left cheek by pushing through your right arm. Then roll across your forehead to the right cheek by pushing through your left arm. Take your time and find a way to roll gently and slowly across your forehead from cheek to cheek so that you can look out at your sides. Notice that each time you push through your arm, you are also moving your rib cage and spine from side to side. Now leave this movement and rest your head and arms in any comfortable position. Stay on your stomach.

Change Your Age Tip: As you do this movement, feel that your arms are providing support for your neck. Imagine that your head is a ball rolling at the end of your spine. As you push your rib cage and spine from side to side with your arms, your head will naturally have to follow. See that your pelvis stays flat on the floor. It's the spine and the upper body that are moving from side to side. If you're rolling across your nose, simply lengthen the back of your neck. The longer you make the back of your neck so that your forehead can be on the floor, the less pressure is exerted on your nose.

5. Put your arms back into a push-up position. Have your hands wide, with your elbows up. This time put your chin on the floor.

6. Now put your forehead on the floor again, but see whether you can rest higher up on your forehead—more toward the hairline than you were before.

Notice what happens in your chest. Now put your chin on the floor, setting it farther away from you than you had it before. Alternate, very slowly, between your forehead and your chin. As you do, move farther up on your forehead each time, as though you wanted to look under yourself, toward your belly. When you set your chin on the floor, set it farther away from your body so that you can look out farther.

As you go back and forth, notice the movement of your chest and lower back. Notice how your legs are involved in the movement.

Now leave this movement and once again rest on your stomach in any comfortable position you can find. If you can't rest on your stomach, then, of course, roll onto your side or your back to rest.

● **Body Intelligence Reminder for Advanced Variations A and B on**
● **Lesson 6:** Don't compete with yourself to do an advanced variation before
● you are ready.

Advanced Variation A on Lesson 6:
REGAINING FULL USE OF YOUR NECK

● **Intention:** To counteract the tendency to slump by making you aware of the relationship of your shoulder blades to your ribs and head. Make sure you have done Lesson 6 before you attempt this posture control lesson.

● **Starting Position:** Lie on your stomach.

1. Lying on your stomach, put your forehead on the floor and place your interlaced hands on the back of your head so that you feel the weight of your hands on the back of your skull, with your nose on the floor. There should be no pressure on your nose; to eliminate any such pressure, all you need to do is lengthen the back of your neck. If the back of your neck is shortened, arch it and you'll find yourself pressing on your nose. If you lengthen your neck, you'll decrease that pressure.

2. With your hands on the back of your head, lift your elbows and then set them down. Do this several times, up and down, and feel which muscles you use. You'll notice that you're using the backs of your shoulders and the muscles between your shoulder blades. For many people, this area tends to be quite weak. This weakness can cause the shoulders to fall forward and the upper part of the body to slump; you may have noticed yourself doing this when you're very tired. This movement will strengthen that area.

3. The next time your elbows are up and you feel that they're level, keep them there. Imagine that from elbow to elbow, through both arms and your interlaced hands, you are a board that is set on top of the back of your head. Now gently push into your head with your right hand and

pull your left elbow to your left, so that your head rolls onto your left cheek. Then push your left hand into the side of your head and roll your head onto your right cheek.

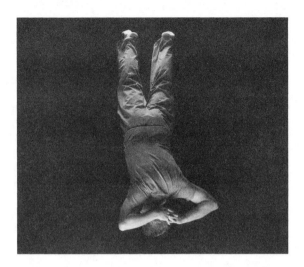

4. Begin to roll across your forehead from cheek to cheek, keeping your elbows as far off the floor as you can. Experiment with how you can keep your elbows off the floor. Roll from cheek to cheek across your forehead and as you do this feel that your arms are moving from side to side while your head rolls almost passively underneath them.

Change Your Age Tip: To decrease the stress and work in your neck, you should feel that, as you roll from one cheek across your forehead to the other cheek, your shoulders and arms are moving from side to side. Your rib cage expands and opens on one side and then closes on the other. The more you put your attention on the work in your upper back, ribs, shoulders, and arms, the less work you'll feel in your neck.

When you roll your head to one side, see whether you can look underneath your arm, out to the side. Keep going that way, always trying to look underneath your elbow. You'll discover a lot of work in the muscles of the lower back, and you'll feel your pelvis working to stabilize and counterbalance the movements of your upper body. Feel free to take a break from the movement if necessary.

Rest. Now roll over and lie on your back, taking a complete rest with your arms and legs long. Give your weight to the floor. Notice the relationship of your head and neck to the floor. Do your neck and shoulders feel any different? Very gently and slowly, see how it feels now to roll your head from side to side.

More Advanced Variation B on Lesson 6:
REGAINING FULL USE OF YOUR NECK

● **Intention:** To counteract the tendency to slump and to develop the brain-muscle connections to raise your head and eyes against gravity.

● **Starting Position:** Lie on your stomach.

1. Interlace your fingers and place them on the floor in front of your face, with your elbows wide apart. Put your forehead on the backs of your interlaced hands.
2. Next, try to lift your head and look out. Do you feel the pressure going down through your hands? Engage more of yourself by feeling your jaw and throat release as you lift your head.
    Practice looking out and turning your head from side to side a few times.
    Rest on your stomach in a comfortable position.
3. Now, could you bend both of your knees so that your feet are aiming toward the ceiling?
    Lift your head again and look out. As you lift your skull, your jaw may come with it. Look around. You have the support of your elbows. Lift up your right leg and set it down.

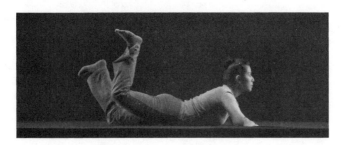

Practice this only a few times until you can feel how to breathe and make it easy.

When you lift your right leg, you'll find it's easier to lift your head.

Then lift your left leg as you lift your head. Slowly alternate lifting your legs as you lift your head.

Rest comfortably on your stomach.

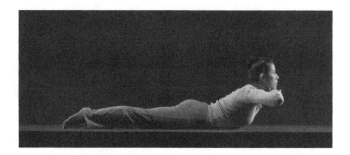

4. Can you bend your knees and interlace your fingers again?

Put your chin down on the back of your interlaced fingers, keeping your elbows wide. Now lift up your arms with your head as if your head and hands were glued together, and look forward. You'll notice that your legs also want to lift and that letting them lift might make it easier for you to lift your head and arms. You'll feel exactly where you have to press against the floor with your belly to support the movement of your back. (These are the ground forces of your trunk being used against the floor to stabilize your back.)

Rest on your stomach for a minute.

5. Now we are going to review an earlier movement to see whether it is easier. Put your hands in a push-up position and rest your forehead on the floor.

Roll your head from side to side, using your body and your arms as the motor.

Roll your head to relax your neck, especially the back of your neck.

6. Roll over onto your back and rest. Do a brief State of the Body Scan. Slowly stand up.

See what has happened to your ability to look left, right, up, and down. Do you feel longer in your back and more open in your chest? Is your sense of the space around you more expansive?

Take a minute to walk around and experience these sensations in your body.

POSITION 1: LYING DOWN ON YOUR SIDE

A favorite sleep position for some people is on their side. It is often a good idea to sleep on your side if you suffer from sleep apnea or if your back hurts when you lie on it for too long.

In these lessons, side-lying is a transitional position from which you will be constantly moving. If you find it hard to lie on one shoulder, or if your hips press into the floor too much, please put extra padding—a blanket will do—where you feel the pressure. If you feel like your head is hanging down to the floor too much and your neck is overstretched, put something under your head—folded towels, for example, or a towel over a book—so that it is slightly elevated.

Lesson 7: A SIMPLE ROLLING LESSON

● **Intention:** To learn a path of least resistance—an easy way to coordinate your whole body into a languid roll.

● **Starting Position:** Lie on your back with your arms and legs long.

1. Very gently, turn your right leg farther to the right, opening the thigh, and let your knee softly bend so that the outside edge of your right foot slides on the floor up toward you. Keep your right leg suspended open to the side for a few seconds before you slide your foot back down the same track it went up. Repeat this movement several times, very slowly, searching for the path of least resistance, as you slide the

outside edge of your foot on the floor. Pausing before you slide your foot up or down gives your brain time to sense things more precisely.

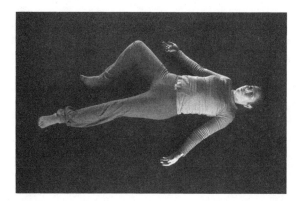

As you slide your foot up and down, release the muscles on the inside and outside of your thigh that do not support the simple action of bending or straightening your hip and knee. Concentrate on releasing the inner muscles of your leg as you perform this movement.

After exploring sliding the edge of your foot up and down the floor, rest your arms and legs long and observe what has changed in the way your leg rests on the floor. Is your leg softer? Is the foot pointing in a different direction than it was earlier? Does your hip feel softer? You might even find that your lower back has released to the floor on the right side.

2. As you slide your right foot up again, reach your left arm across to the right side of your body at the same time.

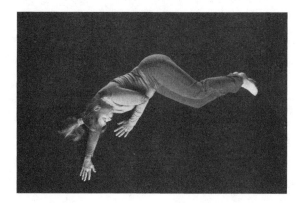

Let your long left leg turn, bend your knee, and slide your relaxed left leg on top of your right leg. You are now lying on your right side with both knees bent and pulled up toward yourself.

To get back to your original position, slide your left leg straight, and then your right leg. Your left arm will cross your body and go back to where it was when you started.

Perform this easy rolling movement a few times until you feel no effort doing it.

Some people may tend to put their arm so close to their body on the side they are rolling toward that the arm is in the way. So pay attention if, for instance, you're rolling to the right—to put your right arm away from your right side.

Feel the timing. Your right leg slides up, your right knee hangs open, your head turns, your left arm reaches across your body, and your left leg sweeps over to the right. These coordinated movements become smooth. You don't need to press against the floor to roll this way. It's as if somebody else is rolling you.

Check your breathing to make sure that you're not stopping your breath or changing its speed at any point.

Stop rolling and rest on your back.

Change Your Age Tip: Most people don't know how to roll their body. Instead, they push themselves against the floor or bend their knee and push themselves over on their standing foot. Some people hold their breath, do a partial sit-up, and lie back down on their side. That's why people feel as if they have to roll uphill. By contrast, this simple lesson is designed to make rolling an easy and pleasurable thing to do.

---

3. For a few moments, practice doing the same thing, still to the right side.

    Then rest again on your back. Imagine doing the same easy rolling movement on the other side. Lie as still as possible on your back as you imagine doing it on the other side.

    Now perform the movement of rolling to the left side.

    Repeat the instructions in Steps 1 and 2 as you roll to the left.

Challenge yourself to make the movement as smooth and easy as you did on the right.

4. This time we are going to add an awareness device. Roll to the right again, but make the movement with increased effort, as if you were acting. Keep yourself tight, not in an exaggerated way but by making yourself stiff in the legs as you roll back and forth and letting your arms cross over your body in an ungainly and mistimed fashion so that your arms are not coordinated with your legs. (When we play-act in this way, we increase the brain activity involved in our movements, and this enables us to become more aware of how we are moving and speeds the learning process.) Now roll again without all this stiffness and feel the difference.

Some people have a habit of holding their breath while they roll. Observe whether you can coordinate the muscular activity of breathing with the muscles required for rolling. Breathing and moving require coordination. Feel that you can roll onto your side and back in one simple breath, inhaling and exhaling each time you roll.

Feel as if you are being poured onto each side and your back.

Rest on your back and take a moment to observe the feelings in your body and how comfortably you are able to breathe.

5. After resting for a while, come to standing.

How do you feel after rolling so easily and performing work with so little effort? Observe whether you like the consequences. Walk around. Do you feel refreshed? What age do you feel now?

Variation on Lesson 7:
SIMPLE ROLLING FROM SIDE-LYING TO SITTING

● **Intention:** To feel a strong connection between your legs and your upper body. You will feel more clearly how your back and pelvis can make you taller.

● **Starting Position:** Lie on your right side again, with your knees and hips bent. Place your right arm in front of yourself and place the palm of your left hand on the floor in front of your chest.

1. Reach your left leg down away from your pelvis as if someone was pulling your leg and roll up onto your right elbow. As your leg reaches long, push through your left hand and right arm and lift your head. When you lift your head, you'll find yourself looking at your left hand. Reverse the motion to return to lying on your right side. Go up and down a few times so that you find yourself rolling up over your elbow enough that your face looks down.

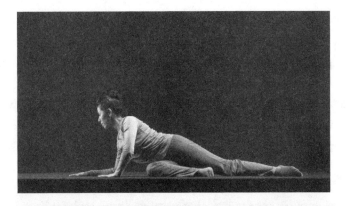

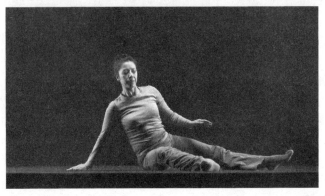

2. If you feel unable to roll up over your elbow, explore different places where you could position your right arm and your left hand. Eventually you'll find a way in which reaching down with your leg and rolling forward with your body will roll you up over your elbow.

3. The next time you reach down with your leg, come to sitting with both hands on the floor. Then straighten both legs and sit for a little

while. You'll end up sitting with your legs a little bit apart, and you'll be able to place your hands behind you.

4. Perform the same movement starting on the left side. If you feel playful, roll from the left side to the right side by coming up through sitting.

Lesson 8: THE MIDDLE OF THE BODY: EXPANDING, REACHING, AND TURNING

● **Intention:** To decrease stress and tightness while increasing the ease of motion in your waist. Stress commonly causes a person to tighten in the middle of the body. This reflex tightness is meant only as a temporary protection during a crisis, but it can become a habit. In this de-aging lesson, you will explore how the movement of the arm or the head requires participation throughout the body if strain is to be avoided. Reaching more easily involves understanding the connection of the arms to the torso and pelvis.

● **Starting Position:** Lie on your left side with your hips and knees bent at right angles and your arms straight out in front of you at chest level. See that the palms and fingers of your hands are resting together and make sure that your elbows are straight.

Change Your Age Tip: If your neck is strained when you lie on your side, put a folded towel under your head so that your neck is supported. If it does not seem possible for both elbows to rest straight, you might need to adjust your side-lying position. If you are rolled slightly forward, your top elbow will be bent. If you are rolled backward, your fingertips won't line up.

---

1. Slowly slide your right palm along your left palm, reaching for the floor in front of you, then slide the left palm over your right hand and forearm. Repeat this motion several times, sliding your right palm forward, then back along your left forearm and upper arm. Feel the texture of your arm and the floor. You will notice that your range of motion expands naturally as you repeat the movement. Think about

where the ability to reach farther comes from. Does your back assist? Does your pelvis move?

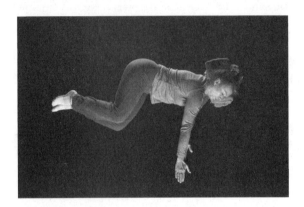

2. The next time you slide your right palm along your left palm and left forearm, continue to slide it all the way across your chest. Make sure you are performing long, lazy movements. Make sure your hand is always touching some part of your body softly and fully. Do not move any farther than you are able to go while still breathing comfortably. You will find it's not worth it to compromise easy, natural breathing. Repeat this movement several times, then rest long and comfortably on your back.

3. This time roll onto your left side in the same position, knees and feet touching, and bring your right hand to cover your forehead, with your elbow pointing straight in the air. Roll your head slowly toward the floor and back, feeling your elbow move through space, until you are facing the ceiling. What happens to your waist? What happens in your ribs? The next time you roll, see whether you can gently bring your elbow all the way toward the floor in front of you. When you roll your head to face the ceiling, can you bring your right elbow all the way toward the floor behind you? Feel the opening in your chest and the movement in your waist. Don't strain to do this motion. Instead, move more slowly and carefully each time. Take a full rest on your side with your elbows and palms together.

4. Glide your right palm slowly against your left palm, moving it forward and then bringing it back toward your chest. Can you bring your right

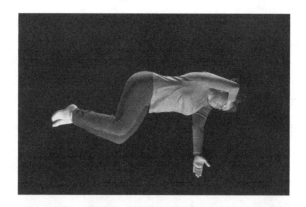

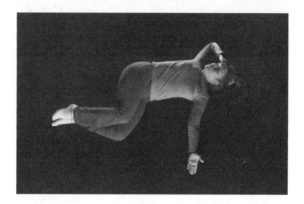

arm all the way across your chest? Can you bring it to your right shoulder? Can you bring it back behind you so that the back of your right
hand is resting on the floor? To do this, allow your knees to separate if
they want to, and feel the movement of your pelvis against the floor.
Repeat this movement several times. Take a full rest on your back.

5. Roll onto your right side with your hips and knees at right angles, your
arms level with your chest and bent at the elbows, and your palms and
fingertips together. Slide your left palm slowly along the right one
onto the floor, then bring it back along your right forearm and upper
arm. Can you bring your left arm across your chest? Is it easier on this
side? Can you bring your left arm behind you so that the back of your
left hand rests on the floor? Rest briefly on your right side with your
fingertips touching.

6. Bring your left hand to your forehead with your palm flat against your forehead and your elbow pointing straight in the air. Roll your head a little bit forward, toward the floor, then back toward the ceiling. Feel the direction of your elbow in the air. Can you sense the inside of your mouth? The back of your right knee? Roll your head gently forward and rest on your side with your left palm against your forehead and your left elbow touching the floor.

7. Roll onto your left side and arrange yourself with your hips and knees at right angles and your arms level with your chest and bent at the elbows. This time, clasp your hands together with your fingers interlocked. Gently slide your right knee forward and backward over your left knee, keeping your ankles and feet together. Don't lift the right knee off the left knee; simply slide it forward, then backward. Let your pelvis and waistline turn while you keep your elbows straight. Can you feel your pelvis clearly rolling? Rest on your side with your palms flat against each other.

8. Now slide your right hand against your left hand toward the floor while sliding your right knee backward. Then do the opposite. As you bring your right hand back, roll your right knee forward.

   Repeat this motion several times until it becomes easier to do this opposition of arm and leg. Make sure you can breathe comfortably. Give yourself time to learn. Rest long and comfortably on your back.

9. Roll onto your right side with your elbows straight in front of you, hands interlocked. Slide your left knee forward and backward against your right knee, using your pelvis and back to help.

   In your own time, repeat these opposing movements of arms and legs. Do not strain—let it happen gently, in its own time.

   Take a long, full rest on your back and observe your comfort on the floor. You may discover that you have lost several years of stressed muscles.

Body Intelligence Reminder: Don't compete with yourself to do an advanced lesson before you are ready.

Lesson 9: CROSSED-ARM, CROSSED-ANKLE FOOT LIFTING—ADVANCED LYING LESSON

Intention: To improve your coordination and sharpen your physical sense of left and right. Your brain will have an opportunity to encounter confusion and solve a puzzle through thinking, sensing, and moving. A little muscle and mind confusion requires your brain to expand.

Starting Position: Lie on your back, bend both knees, and put both feet in a standing position.

1. Bring your left knee toward your left shoulder and place your right hand on top of your left foot. Keeping your right thumb together with your fingers, hold on to the outside edge of your left foot. If it's not possible to hold on to your left foot without straining, hold your left ankle, your big toe, or your pant leg—whatever is most comfortable.

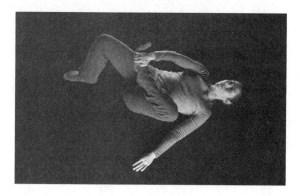

Lift your right knee toward your right shoulder and reach your left hand to the outside edge of your right foot and hold on to it in the same way. You will have two hands simultaneously holding on to two feet, with your right ankle crossed on top of your left ankle.

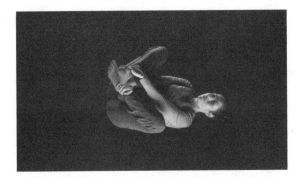

Can you breathe in this position? Become familiar with the feeling of holding on to your feet in this configuration. Feel and see how your feet are crossed and your hands are uncrossed.

2. As you continue to hold on to your feet, lift both of them up into the air and uncross them.

Your arms will be crossed, left over right, and your knees will be bent. As you lift your feet and slightly straighten your legs, your arms will cross even more.

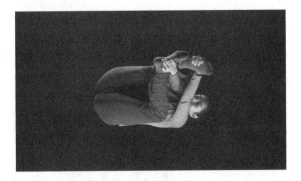

Let go of your feet and take a full rest on your back, with your arms and legs long.

3. Arrange yourself by holding on to your feet, in exactly the same way you just did in Step 1.

Lift your feet into the air again.

As you continue to hold on to your feet, uncross your ankles and re-cross them so that your left ankle is over your right ankle. Roll on your back from side to side and continue to uncross and recross your legs and arms as you roll. Continue to practice this as long as it feels comfortable.

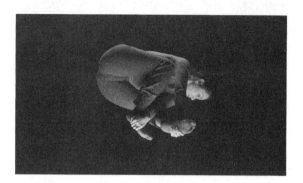

Pause and rest.

Rest on your back, with your arms and legs long, and take a State of the Body Scan of your back against the floor. While you're lying on the floor with your eyes closed, simply imagine doing some of these movements.

4. Play with this movement again for a few minutes and practice what you used in your imagination. Refer to the instructions and photo in Step 3 to help you recall the felt sense of the movement.

For your own reference, return to just holding on to your feet with crossed ankles and see how much easier it is to perform the first movement.

Rest on your back with your arms and legs long and feel your body against the floor. Notice whether you have more contact with your back and your legs against the floor.

5. Slowly come to standing. Does your spine feel longer? Maybe you've reduced compression in your spine. Do your hips feel younger? Do you feel taller?

This is an age-changing coordination challenge.

POSITION 2: SITTING

Sitting has become one of the most common activities performed by humans. This amazing imposition on the human body is now considered a necessity for both work and rest. A lot of people don't realize that sitting puts more pressure on their spinal disks than standing does. That is why some people hurt when they sit in chairs. When we walk, we constantly vary the pressure on our disks. So, in this section, we will learn to create a more mobile way of sitting.

POSITION 2: SITTING ON THE FLOOR

Lesson 10: TURNING FROM YOUR PELVIS

- **Intention:** To develop and strengthen the pelvic and core muscles of your body and free up your hips and spine.

- **Starting Position:** Sit on the floor with your legs long in front of yourself.

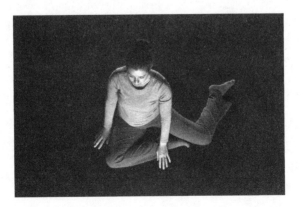

1. Turn your pelvis to the right and keep turning until your knees start to bend. Let your knees bend and your feet slide so that you are side-sitting with your hands in an easy place on the floor to the right.

2. Turn your pelvis back to the middle and feel how your legs straighten in front of yourself again.

3. Then turn your pelvis to the left and feel how your knees and feet can follow your pelvis by sliding toward yourself. Let your knees straighten when you are in the center.

   Repeat the motion of turning the pelvis with the knees and arms several times.

   You'll discover that there's a coherent movement from turning the pelvis to the right, putting your hands on the floor, bending your knees, while sliding your feet closer to yourself.

   There's another coherent movement in turning your pelvis forward and straightening your legs out in front of you.

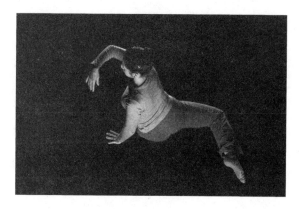

4. Next, try alternating turning from one side to the other. Feel how your legs straighten in the middle.

   As you turn your pelvis to the right, let your legs pull toward yourself and let your arms swing to the right while your head turns to look over your right shoulder.

   Then turn your pelvis to the left by letting your legs go straight, turning to the left side, and letting your head look over your left shoulder. Do this movement a few times until it becomes smoother.

   Some people enjoy turning like this several times. Try practicing the movement only enough times to make it lighter. Be cautious if you have difficulties with your hips, knees, or back. It's a useful and good movement to learn, but your body may need some time to adjust to it. It's better to do this movement only a little bit if side-sitting is a strained position for you.

If you're comfortable with this movement, vary the speed and go side to side a little faster. Go as fast as your arms will swing, with your pelvis and legs following. See that your pelvis can turn at the speed of your arms and that your legs can follow.

Rest briefly in side-sitting or with your legs in front of yourself. Then rest on your back and do a State of the Body Scan.

Lesson 11: DEVELOPING LONGER HAMSTRINGS THE EASY WAY

● **Intention:** To learn comfortably how to lengthen your hamstrings so that the muscles can retain their length. The hamstrings are important because they flex the knee; when we walk, the hamstrings pull the foot backward at the knee, while also contributing, along with the gluteal muscles of the buttocks, to extending our hips. The hamstrings contribute to stabilizing our knees when we push, as in jumping. Since these are very common activities, the hamstrings tend to get short and tight. Most exercise programs encourage stretching muscles like the hamstrings, but I want to encourage you to lengthen your muscles permanently without stretching.

Do a State of the Body Scan. Lie on your back with your legs long and feel the space between the backs of your legs and the floor. The tighter your hamstrings, the bigger the space will be. Your two legs might feel different from each other.

● **Starting Position:** Sit with your left leg bent in back of you and your right leg straight out in front. Make sure your left foot is in a comfortable place behind you, with your left knee slightly forward. If this position is uncomfortable, bring your left foot in front of yourself, near your crotch, and let your left knee hang open toward the floor. You can lean on your right hand for support.

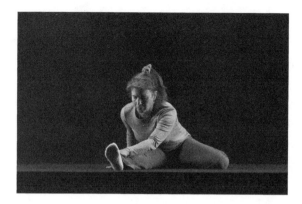

1. Put your left hand on the outside of your right thigh and slowly massage your right leg by kneading and rubbing the muscles, sliding over them with your hand. Massage in long, slow strokes down toward your ankle. Make sure that your hand is in constant contact with all sides of your leg and that you breathe fully. Massage your leg until you feel the muscles releasing comfortably.

    Pause and rest your legs.

Change Your Age Tip: Feel the texture of your right leg as well as its shape, as though you were exploring it for the first time. Make long, steady strokes down toward your right ankle and back toward your hip. The secret of this movement lies in how smoothly and easily you can move back and forth. Pay no attention to how far you're going. Notice that if you let your shoulder release and allow your body to turn to the right, it's quite easy to go farther.

---

2. Put your right leg out in front of you again, with a straight knee. Put your leg at a different angle to your trunk by placing it a little more to the right or left. Begin massaging the inside of your right leg with your left hand and experience how you rock back and forth on your pelvis as you reach with your left shoulder and your head. If you happen to touch your foot, fine. If you can only go to just below your knee, that's also fine. Let your right knee bend whenever it wants to so that the right leg is soft and can adjust easily to your massaging. See whether

you can massage some part of your foot, perhaps playing with your toes. Allow your knee to bend to help you. After you feel you've massaged your leg well enough, rest on your back and feel the difference in your two legs.

3. Roll to one side and sit again. This time put your right foot in back of yourself and your left leg straight in front, so that you're sitting like a mirror image of the previous position. Use your left hand for support on the floor and begin massaging your left leg thoroughly with your right hand.

Change Your Age Tip: You'll have more weight on your left hip now. Remember that if the position is difficult, you can sit with your right foot near your crotch, with your right knee hanging open. Let your head and neck relax completely as you rock back and forth toward and away from your foot. Every so often, play with your toes, allowing your left knee to bend so that you can do so. You may never before in your life have taken the time to slowly and carefully massage your legs. Often we know nothing about our bodies until something hurts or goes wrong. Only then do we look at ourselves carefully and with concern.

Rest on your back again and take time to feel the change.

4. Sit up again, this time leaning on your hands comfortably in back of you, with your legs straight in front of you. Toss your legs wide apart, then bring them back again, as though you were opening and closing a pair of scissors. Do this several times. Forcing the legs to open beyond a natural and comfortable width for you is not the point of this movement. The act of "tossing" your legs apart will allow them to land in an unforced and natural position for your body.

Now leave your legs wide apart wherever they go easily. Put both hands on your right leg near the hip and begin to massage down the leg toward your foot in long, languid strokes. Let yourself breathe out as you go down your leg.

5. The next time your hands return to your hip, let them slide over your belly to your left hip, and begin to massage down your left leg and

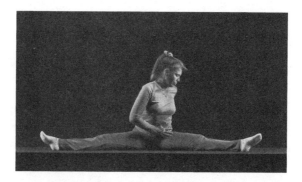

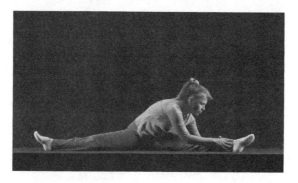

back again. Think of yourself as a sculptor, shaping your legs as you massage. As you go down one leg and then the other, think of passing your hands across your body, as if you were sculpting the connection of your legs to your torso. Go in a smooth and steady motion.

Change Your Age Tip: Let your head, neck, and shoulders be soft and relaxed as you massage. Let your pelvis rock from side to side on the floor. Every so often, vary what you do with your feet by pulling them back and keeping your knees straight. Remember, your goal is to let the movement be sensual, as if you were making a sensual sculpture of your lower body. Every so often let your knees go soft and bend as they need to.

Rest on your back with your arms and legs long and observe how close your legs and back are to the floor. Perhaps you've created softer, younger muscles by lengthening them without stress.

Lesson 12: OILING YOUR HIPS THE EASY WAY

● **Intention:** To learn a fun and exhilarating way to release stiffness in your hips, knees, and lower back.

● **Starting Position:** Lie on your back with your arms and legs long. Take a moment to observe your contact with the floor. Focus your attention inside your body.

1. Come to sitting with your knees bent so that the bottoms of your feet are standing on the floor. Close your eyes and, with your left hand, reach around the outside of your left knee, holding on to the outside edge of your left foot, near your toes, keeping your thumb together with your fingers. Lift your foot in the air and set it down a few times. Feel what your pelvis and lower back need to do to help you. Feel free to use your right hand on the floor for support.

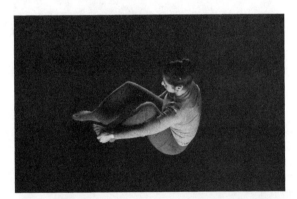

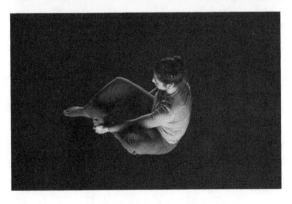

The next time you lift your left foot up and set it down, have your knee cross underneath your arm so that it flips to the outside of your left arm as you set the foot down. Then the next time you lift your foot up, set it down and flip your left knee to the inside. Do this movement slowly several times so that you can feel what happens in your hip joint to create this turning of the knee under your arm.

Rest on your back with your arms and legs long. Take time to notice the difference between the two sides of your body. Which side feels younger?

2. Come to sitting and hold on to your left foot, arranging yourself exactly the same way as before. Lift your foot up and set it down somewhere else on the floor. In fact, lift it up and set it down in as many different places on the floor as you can find. Be exploratory and playful. Cross your foot to the other side of your body and find a couple of ways to set your foot in back of yourself or even raise it above your head.

3. Now arrange yourself similarly, this time with your right hand reaching around the outside of your right knee and holding on to the outside edge of your right foot. As in Step 1, explore how to flip your knee back and forth under your right elbow. Take the time to feel this carefully. Can your right knee pass under your right elbow and shoulder without making any contact with your arm? Are you still breathing?

4. Sit again with your right hand holding the outside edge of your right foot. As in Step 2, explore all the places you can touch on the floor around your body with this foot. Rest on your back with your legs long and enjoy your contact with the floor.

5. Come to sitting with both of your knees pointing to your right and both of your feet to the left. This will put you in a side-sitting position, with your left foot just in back of you on the floor and your right foot near your left knee. In fact, your left knee will probably be touching the bottom of your right foot.

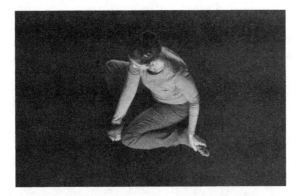

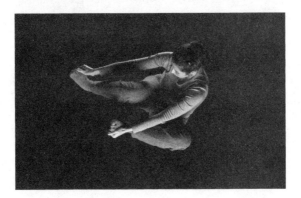

At the same time, hold on to the outside edge of your left foot with your left hand and the outside edge of your right foot with your right hand, with your fingers and thumbs together curling around the bottoms of your feet. Lift both feet from the floor and simultaneously flip both of your knees under both of your elbows. As your knees get straighter, come to side-sitting in a mirror of your starting position. Your knees are now to the left and your feet to the right, with your left foot touching or near your right thigh.

Change Your Age Tip: As you move your feet from one side of your body to the other, in side-sitting, you will experience yourself rolling on your pelvis from side to side, and you will need to lift your feet high in the air for your knees to flip under your elbows. Make sure that you don't strain or hold your breath. Work to make the movement easy.

Take your feet and knees from side to side this way, several times. Make it easier each time. Rest on your back with your arms and legs long.

6. Return to side-sitting. Choose your favorite side. Hold on again with both hands to both outside edges of your feet. Once again, you'll be changing to side-sitting on the other side by flipping your knees under your arms, but this time try to do it by sliding your feet on the floor the entire time as your knees change from side to side.

Rest on your back and do a State of the Body Scan, noticing the changes in your back. When you get up to walk, notice whether your legs and back have more freedom.

POSITION 2: SITTING IN A CHAIR

Since sitting in a chair puts more pressure on the disks of the spine, many people have to stand frequently to relieve muscular contractions, which are harder to notice in a static position like sitting. Therefore, if you sit for long periods of time, it is extremely important to have good, stress-free posture that enables you to perform tasks comfortably. The lessons in this section will help if your job involves sitting at a desk for prolonged periods of time.

For these lessons, please sit in a chair that is flat and firm. An ordinary wooden chair or a chair with light padding would be best. The flatter the surface the better. Make sure the chair has no armrests. The height of the chair should allow your hips to be as high as or higher than your knees. Do not do these lessons on a sofa, in an armchair, or on a chair that is low to the floor.

Lesson 13: CHAIR PLAY

● **Intention:** To develop more flexible ideas about how to relate to a chair so as to create a much more flexible body. Many people have overly rigid ideas about how they should sit in a chair. Remember how a child relates to a chair and all the different ways in which children move their bodies in relationship to a chair.

● **Starting Position:** Sit near the front of your chair. Make sure both of your feet are solidly on the floor, with your feet and knees well apart.

1. As you sit, can you feel your two sitting bones (the bones on the bottom of your pelvis on each side)? Observe, without making changes, which sitting bone bears most of your weight—the right or the left? You can sit on several areas of your sitting bones from the front to the back and anywhere in between.

   Roll your pelvis toward the back of your sitting bones, then roll toward the front of your sitting bones. Does your upper torso move forward or backward?

2. Place the palm of your right hand on your lower back and the palm of your left hand on the top of your head. Make sure you feel both feet solidly on the floor.

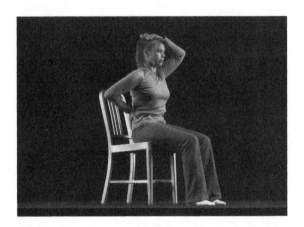

Move your lower back into your right hand by rolling your pelvis on the chair and notice that you're sitting on the back part of your sitting bones. Then roll your pelvis until you feel your back hollow into an arch and notice that you're sitting on the front part of your sitting bones. As you do this movement back and forth, observe the change in the height of your head. Do this movement several times until the feeling is clear. Rest with your arms down. Are you sitting more on your right side?

Change Your Age Tip: If it is too difficult to put the palm of your hand on your back, put the back of your hand there. Your only effort should be in sensing the movement. Feel your vertebrae with your fingertips and your muscles with your hand.

3. Repeat Step 2 with the palm of your left hand on your lower back and the palm of your right hand on your head. Which side is easier? Which side makes you raise and lower your height the most? Which side makes it easier to hollow your back? Rest and observe. Which side bears more weight?

4. Sit on the right side of your chair so that the right side of your pelvis is unsupported and your right buttock and sitting bone are completely off the chair. Only the left side of your buttock will remain on the chair. Put your right hand on your waistline as you would in a casual way, with your fingers spread toward your stomach and your thumb in the back.

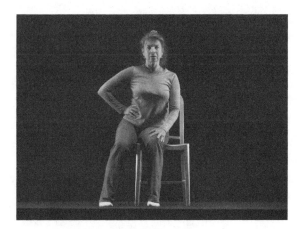

Lower and raise the right side of your pelvis so that it goes below the level of the chair and then above it. Can you feel the right side of your waistline lengthening and shortening? If you put your left hand on top of your head at the same time, can you feel the connection between the movement of your pelvis and your entire spine and neck? Repeat this movement several times and then rest, sitting back in your chair on both sitting bones, and notice if you feel them more clearly.

Change Your Age Tip: Make sure your feet and legs are fairly wide apart and observe how your right leg assists the right side of your pelvis by pushing your heel into the floor so that you can use ground forces through your legs. You might want to experiment by lifting your right heel from the floor as you lower the right side of your pelvis.

5. Repeat Step 4 on the other side by having your left sitting bone completely off the chair and only your right buttock on the chair, with your left hand on your waist and your right hand on the top of your head. Make sure that your legs are wide apart. Is this side more or less fluid than the other side? Rest sitting back in your chair and notice how you are resting on your sitting bones now.

6. Sit facing the back of your chair. Lean your folded arms on the top of the back of the chair, with your pelvis near the front of the chair. Roll your pelvis forward to hollow your back, then backward to curve it. Try this movement with your forehead resting on your folded arms still on the back of the chair. Can you also rock your pelvis from side to side in this position, pushing through one foot while lifting one side of the pelvis and then the other? Try this both with your head looking out and with your forehead resting on your forearms.

7. Put your hands on your knees and put your chest against the back of the chair, with your head looking down and your eyes closed. Roll your pelvis forward, pushing your belly out toward the back of the chair and then backward, holding it in as your spine curves away from your chair. Let your belly push forward and backward in harmony with the movement of your spine and pelvis until it becomes easy to feel how your breathing can assist the motion. Rest leaning on the back of your chair.

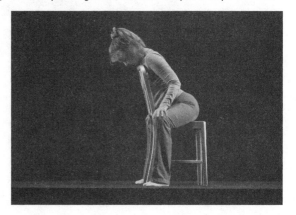

Change Your Age Tip: For many people with difficulties in their middle or lower back, it is much easier to sit facing the back of a chair because this position provides support and requires opening the hips. This lesson and any of the movements in it are useful to perform whenever stress accumulates from sitting.

Lesson 14: THE SITTING AND TURNING DANCE

● **Intention:** To further explore how you sit in a chair and provide you with greater core muscle strength, better balance, and improved range of scanning.

● **Starting Position:** Sit in your chair with plenty of room around yourself. If you have a mat, put your chair toward the back of your mat, not on your mat. Sit so that your back isn't leaning against the back of the chair. Have your feet on the floor next to each other, a little bit apart.

1. Notice how you are sitting in the chair. While you're sitting, turn your head from side to side and observe which side is easier.

2. Lift up the left side of your pelvis and "walk" it forward. You'll have to push through your left leg to lift the left side of your pelvis, then begin to inch it forward.

   Now do the same thing with the right side. Walk left and right a few times. Now do this movement without lifting your feet off the floor.

   Can you walk both the left side and the right side of your pelvis backward? Walk one side back and then the other.

   Then go a little farther back, but keep your feet on the floor. This can be the hardest part.

   As you are doing this with your pelvis, make sure you really use ground forces through your feet to assist the movement.

3. Begin to walk a couple of steps forward on your sitting bones. Then walk a couple of steps backward, still keeping your feet on the floor.

   Come to the middle in a place that feels neutral to you.

   As a measure of your orientation, look around yourself again. Notice whether it's easier to scan the room, turning from side to side.

Maybe you can see farther around yourself, as if you're taking in more of the environment, with an increased awareness of the space around you. Waking up deep pelvic and core muscles with new movements can affect sensations in the head and face. Some people may find that their face feels larger as well.

4. Next, with your head up and able to scan, walk your feet on the floor so that you can turn your pelvis and sit with your feet on the right side of your chair.

    Then walk yourself back. You are turning on your chair. You may be able to get back and forth in only a couple of steps.

    Pause.

    Then walk your pelvis to the left side.

    Now go from side to side so that you turn completely to the right side of the chair and then completely to the left, almost spinning your pelvis in the chair.

    When you come to the middle again, pause.

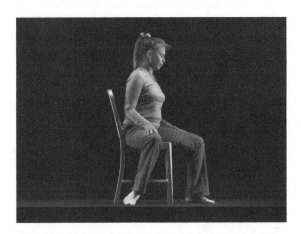

The next movement might make you a little dizzy, so be careful. Rest when you need to and keep breathing.

5. Again, using your feet, walk your pelvis left and right completely. Turn your head to look over your left shoulder while simultaneously turning your pelvis to the right. Then, while turning your pelvis to the left, simultaneously turn your head to look over your right shoulder.

Keep going side to side so that you're continuously looking in the opposite way your pelvis is turning.

Come to the middle again and rest. You can rest any way you want to, leaning back into your chair or not. Turn your head to each side and feel if you can see farther.

● *Body Intelligence Reminder for Advanced Variation on Lesson 14:* Don't compete with yourself to do an advanced variation before you are ready. Remember to practice this lesson slowly, making sure that you don't force yourself to achieve something for which you haven't established a feeling or a felt sense.

Advanced Variation on Lesson 14:
THE SITTING AND TURNING DANCE

● **Intention:** To give you the fullest use of your body as you spin around in your chair and learn to use your hips and back in ways you might not have explored or practiced in many years.

● **Starting Position:** Sit in your chair with plenty of room around yourself.

1. In Lesson 14, we walked and spun from one side of the chair to the other. Another way to continue this movement is to walk all the way around your chair after you find a way to swing your legs over the back of your chair to the other side and continue to pivot your pelvis around in a full circle.

2. You can lift one leg at a time over the back of the chair if you want the movement to be easier. Do that a few times. Keep going around to the right in a full circle. You'll discover that you can move your trunk to keep going in one direction a few times.

   Pause and rest in the middle of your chair. If you find it too difficult to balance, use your hands for support. You will be more aware of the space around yourself.

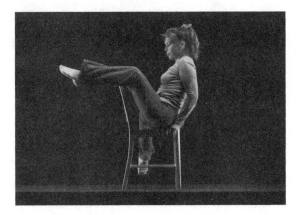

3. Now walk to the left, all the way around your chair. Again, swing your legs one at a time over the back of the chair. Notice the space around yourself as you move. Let your head keep scanning.

Change Your Age Tip: See how quickly you can go around in one direction and how few steps it takes to spin all the way around your chair. Notice whether it's easier to turn completely around on one side compared to the other. You will discover something you probably have never known: the side you can move fastest to in sitting. You can go in a circle as many times as you want. Be playful with it.

Stop, rest, and observe how you are sitting and how expansive the space feels around you. Movements like spinning around in your chair in unusual ways not only make you feel more expansive but also affect your brain by forging new neurons and new connections, which are made when we approach old habitual movements like sitting in a chair in new and playful ways.

Did this playful and novel movement make you feel younger?

Lesson 15: MOVING FROM THE CHAIR TO THE FLOOR AND RETURNING

● **Intention:** To learn an easy and interesting way to move from sitting in a chair to the floor and then back up again.

This lesson is particularly transforming for those who have a fear of falling. One of the most significant changes that occurs as we age is that we begin to be afraid of falling. Many parents—and certainly grandparents—feel too stiff, old, or heavy to get on the floor easily and play with their kids or grandkids or rumble with their dogs. Many people don't get on the floor because it takes so much effort to get up again. This lesson is an important one for people who can't fully admit that they have a hard time getting down on the floor and back up again.

● **Starting Position:** Start by sitting toward the front part of your chair.

1. Place your right hand on the chair for support. Move your left knee and hip forward, keeping your left foot in place on the floor. Your left buttock will come slightly off the chair, and you will end up swiveling toward the right side. Reverse the movement by swiveling back to sit fully on the chair. Go back and forth this way a few times. The next time your left buttock comes off the chair, place your left knee gently on the floor.

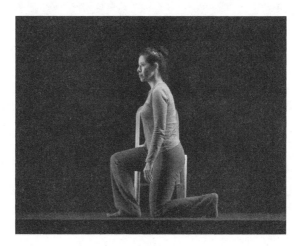

Now you are facing toward the right, solidly standing on your right foot, your right hand is on the chair, wherever it can best support you, and your left knee is kneeling on the floor.

Change Your Age Tip: Don't immediately focus your eyes on the floor—a lot of the fear of falling is stimulated by staring at the floor. Instead, simply feel with your feet that the floor is there.

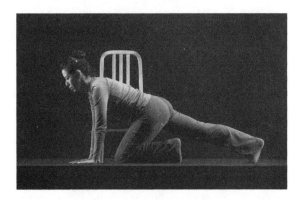

2. Next, place your hands on the floor in front of you, simultaneously sliding your right leg directly in back of yourself.

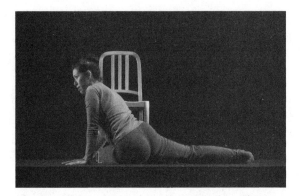

3. Now slowly lower your left hip toward the floor. Your right leg will remain long and relatively straight.

4. Next, get up from this position by lifting your pelvis up over your legs and arms and bringing your right knee forward until you are on all fours. You'll feel how your head and spine move forward to help your pelvis lift from the floor.

5. Keeping both hands on the floor, move your pelvis back as if to sit on your heels, but don't sit on your heels. Instead, move your pelvis off to

the left side and sit on your left buttock. You may need to move your left foot out of the way so you can sit more comfortably.

The goal is to sit on the floor comfortably. Move from sitting to all fours, and vice versa, until the movement feels easily reversible. The next time you are on all fours, pause for a moment.

6. Next, stand on your right foot again. You can place your right hand on the chair to help yourself stand on your right foot. Use your right hand, right foot, and left toes to push into the floor as you bow slightly forward with your trunk and slide your left buttock onto the chair. Basically you swivel on your feet and buttock as you turn to the left. The invisible yet essential ingredient to getting back on the chair smoothly and easily is the bowing and turning of the trunk. If you keep your trunk erect, you will need very strong legs to push you up to sitting. This is a challenging movement for your brain to read, feel, and formulate into action, but don't give up—play with it a few times step by step.

Now come back up and sit on the chair.

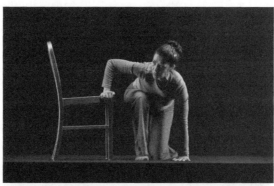

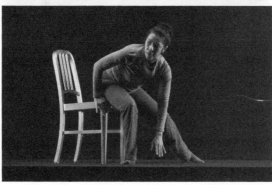

7. Imagine the movements you just performed as if you were actively experiencing them while you remain seated in your chair.

8. Now return to the floor by sliding your left knee and hip forward. When you return to the chair, reread these instructions and revisualize yourself doing the movement.

9. While sitting, close your eyes and visualize yourself performing the entire movement on the other side, with your right knee reaching down to the floor.

Change Your Age Tip: You might find the movement easier to perform if you imagine it well in real time or slower than real time. Research from the fields of both rehabilitation and high-performance athletics has proven that the ability to imagine movement is one of life's great enablers.

Imagine the first movement as your right buttock comes off the chair and your right knee goes down to the floor. Can you feel the friction of your clothes against the chair and how much your head and shoulders turn? Which side of your pelvis do you lean on most heavily? How relaxed is your jaw, and how easy is your breathing? Feel the texture of the floor as you progressively settle your knee on it. Remember to stay seated and imagine this movement through your mind's eye. You might even feel your brain expanding as you project your way through the movement. If you want, physically perform the movement on the right side.

Rest in a sitting position and observe how you are able to organize yourself in the chair. How closely did your movement match your imagination?

As you sit resting, appreciate your sense of space. You may have your eyes closed, but observe that you can notice space around you more. As you look around, scanning the room, notice how thoroughly you can turn and how much of your body is involved. How much younger did you get by doing this? For many people it has been years since they moved in a chair as easily as we have in this section.

Variation on Lesson 15:
MOVING FROM THE CHAIR TO THE
FLOOR AND RETURNING

● **Intention:** To help you gracefully and lightly roll up over your bones from the floor to sitting in a chair. You will reinforce your capacity to move without anxiety or a fear of falling. It's empowering to get up and down from the floor in a variety of ways. You'll feel lighter and more agile, like an airplane that's been de-iced.

● **Starting Position:** Lie on your back, with your arms and legs long, in front of your chair, slightly to the left side of the chair.

1. Roll over onto your right side by bending your knees to the right and reaching with your left hand across your body to the floor.

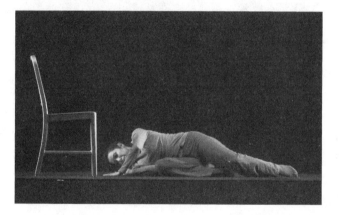

2. Reach with your left leg down away from your pelvis, as if someone were pulling your leg, and roll up onto your right elbow until you are sitting on your right hip with both hands on the floor.
3. Raise your pelvis above your knees as you straighten both arms and lift your head. You should find yourself on all fours.
4. Adjust your position on your hands and knees so that you are near your chair and can place your left hand on the front of the chair.

5. Place your left hand on the left side of your chair as you stand on your left foot on the floor. Push down with your left hand, left foot, and right toes as you turn to the right and sit on your chair.

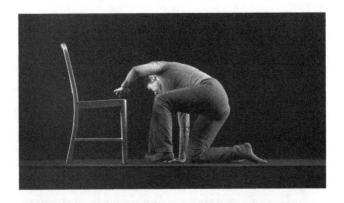

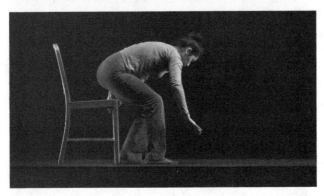

Feel that you could reverse the movement at any point and return to the floor. Go back and forth several times.

Rest by sitting in the chair.

6. Imagine going down and up from the floor. The next time you imagine going down, go all the way down to lying on your back. Imagine doing this on both sides. Not only will this movement melt your old habits, but it will also enable you to create new movements by expanding your physical imagination and adding new neurons to your brain. You might even find that it's good exercise to go down to the

floor and onto your back, then return to sitting—something you could practice on both sides every day. Feel free to invent your own variations, as long as how you do them is clear to you.

Change Your Age Tip: For practice, try going at various speeds so that you can go up and down from the floor without bumping. Feel how smooth the movement can be and how light you can make your return to the chair. Practice on the other side.

This movement is very stimulating to the inner ear, and sometimes we need to take time to adjust to that. When you increase your speed, you might find yourself getting dizzy. If so, simply rest sitting in the chair for a while. Eventually the exercise will strengthen your vestibular system and improve your balance. You'll find yourself becoming less concerned about approaching and leaving the floor.

Lesson 16: JUMP-SITTING IN A CHAIR

● **Intention:** To help you discover an ideal, alert sitting posture. Sitting is part of a movement that goes from squatting to jumping. To gracefully move from sitting through standing into jumping, then return to sitting, would be a sign of good coordination and bodily control. After this lesson, you will be able to sit while fully using your hips and legs and with such good balance in your spine that your muscles will work with less strain.

Better balance eliminates the need to use your arms to push off on a chair as you stand up. This tendency to rely on the arms is a sign of aging as people forget how to use the muscles in their legs and don't trust the balance of their trunk and hips when they go from sitting to standing.

One of the best ways to get out of a chair easily to standing is to sit as if you were preparing yourself to jump out of the chair. You will learn the ideal position for your feet in order to stand up from sitting in a chair.

● **Starting Position:** Sit in the center of a firm, comfortable chair with no arm supports and place both feet in front of yourself in a comfortable place where you know you would put your feet if you were to stand up.

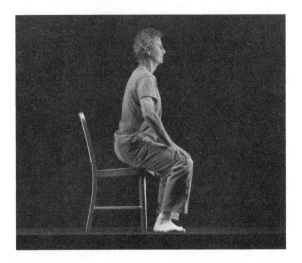

1. Pushing your feet down into the floor, can you lift your pelvis slightly off the chair—only enough to be able to slide a piece of paper out from under yourself? Now set your pelvis down. Feel that each time you lift your pelvis up slightly and lower it down, you need to use only your legs and some deep muscles of your abdomen and back. Rearrange the position of your feet and the distance from your feet to your pelvis until this movement becomes extremely easy. Pause.

2. Now, can you lift your pelvis enough to bounce yourself like a ball in your chair? Continue bouncing your pelvis forward in the chair toward your feet and then backward toward the back of the chair. Let it be a light, quick bounce. Maybe you can bounce all the way from the front of the chair to the back of the chair in one bounce.

3. Now can you bounce your pelvis from one side of the chair to the other, turning as you go?

Change Your Age Tip: Practice bouncing on your chair every day to activate the deep core muscles in your hips and legs and in your abdomen and back.

Advanced Variation on Lesson 16:
JUMP-SITTING ON THE FLOOR

● **Intention:** To wake up and revitalize some of the deep muscles you need to perform common movements that you do all day, such as rising from sitting to standing, bending over and standing up, walking up the stairs or a hill, and getting off the floor to stand. When these muscles are fully in use in this playful way, you'll find that your posture is easier to change and many ordinary activities are easier to perform.

● **Starting Position:** Sit on the floor and bend both of your knees so that you can comfortably put both of your feet in a standing position in front of yourself. Place your hands in back of yourself so that you have a little support.

1. Lift your pelvis slightly off the floor—just enough to be able to slide a piece of paper under yourself. Then set your pelvis down.

    Feel what happens in your shoulders each time you lift your pelvis. How can you position your hands and arrange your posture to make the movement easier?

2. The next time you lift your pelvis, move it a little forward, toward your feet.

3. The next time you lift your pelvis, move it a little backward, toward your hands.

4. Then, the next time, move your pelvis a little bit to the right. Then to the left. And then to the middle.

    As you bounce your pelvis up and down a few times, keep it light—don't smack the floor. Try putting your arms in different positions so that your shoulders feel safe when you lift your pelvis.

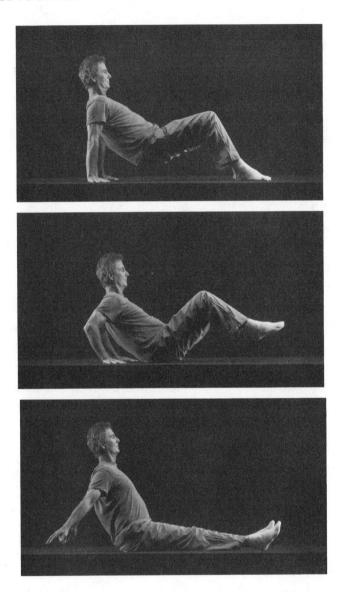

5. Let's play a little game. Lift your hands from the floor just a little bit
   and then place them on the floor. Lift your pelvis from the floor again
   and then set it down. Lift your feet from the floor and then set them
   down. Alternate lifting your hands, pelvis, and feet, hands, pelvis,
   feet. Do this only a few times until you can feel how to make the
   movement lighter.

POSITION 3: KNEELING

So much of the early use of our body to propel us through the world starts against the ground in kneeling and crawling positions. Most of us first become aware of our coordination and certainly the stability of our limbs in relation to our trunk when we're on our knees. Since some people do not enjoy pressure on their knees or wrists, we will begin this position with the Baby Alligator. We'll explore various altitudes of kneeling and learn how to get from the floor up to our knees lightly and easily . . . with no thumping or falling.

Lesson 17: BABY ALLIGATOR

● **Intention:** To help you regain years of mobility in your shoulders and spine and in the movements of your head and neck. As our breathing habits become more formed, it's of great benefit to perform movements that require our ribs and all the muscles of our trunk and neck to regain dexterity. After this lesson, you will experience standing and walking differently. These movements of your shoulder blades will strongly counteract the tendency to slump and to let your shoulders go forward and your chest to drop as you age. Developmentally, most of us performed a version of this lesson when we were babies as our brains prepared us for kneeling, crawling, and ultimately standing and walking.

Do a State of the Body Scan. Lie down on your back and feel your contact with the floor. Stretch out your arms and legs. Put your hands down at your sides.

If you close your eyes, you'll be able to get a better feel for how you're resting on the floor. Notice which of your shoulder blades seems flatter, lower to the floor, more spread out, or wider. Is there a difference in the size of your two hips? One side of your pelvis may also feel flatter or larger—or is it simply pressed more to that side? What is the highest point of your body from the floor? If the ceiling were to lower down and touch the highest point of your body, what part of your body would the ceiling come in contact with first—your nose, chest, stomach, pelvis, or toes? Once you've decided, drop an imaginary line from that highest point straight through your body to the floor. See where this line would come out on your back side.

● **Starting Position:** Roll over onto your stomach. Let your legs be comfortably apart. Put your left hand down to your side, near your hip, and turn your face to look toward the right so that you can see your right arm straight out, at the height of your shoulder.

1. Now bend your right elbow and stand your right hand, as if you were going to do a push-up, with your right elbow in the air. Feel that hand in a firm place on the floor. Since your head is turned to that side, you can see your hand easily and see that there is a distance between your right shoulder and your right hand, so that if you were to drop a line from the inside of your right elbow straight down to the floor, your hand would be farther away from your shoulder than that line. Make sure you have a sizable gap between your right hand and shoulder.

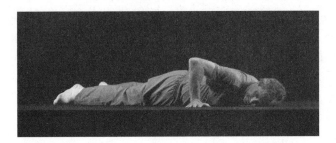

2. Lift your right shoulder toward the ceiling, then set it back down, making sure you set the shoulder back down completely so the muscles can rest. Go back and forth this way a few times. Feel how your shoulder slides back toward your spine, then slides forward away from your spine. The next time you lift your shoulder, push down with your hand and straighten your right elbow, making sure your hand stays in the same place. Feel how your shoulder slides even farther back toward your spine. Notice that the farther back it slides, the more your elbow can straighten. Do this a few times. Rest on your stomach with your head in a comfortable position.

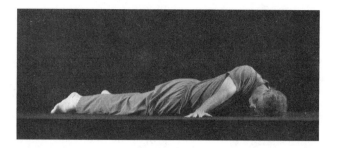

3. Now explore the optimal place to put your right hand, so that you feel some challenge to straighten your right elbow. Your hand could be closer or farther away from your shoulder—in a place that makes the movement neither too easy nor too hard.

4. Now stand your right hand the best distance away from yourself to enable your elbow to straighten. Aim your fingers to the right and spread them wide apart, so that you can feel your whole hand and all of your fingers on the floor. With your elbow pointing directly toward the ceiling, continue to glide your shoulder blade toward and away from your spine. Make sure your hand doesn't move but stays in the spot you chose for it. Keep your fingers pointing away from yourself and your hand spread wide, as if you had a claw. Rest for a moment with your arm down.

Change Your Age Tip: In this lesson, whenever you move your arm, your shoulder and arm, or your leg and hip, make sure that your rib cage remains soft and that you can breathe easily.

---

5. Stand your right hand again—with your fingers pointing away—and roll your right hip off the floor. Now draw your right knee up so that the inside of your right leg is on the floor. Then slide your right knee back down. Do this a few times. As you slide your knee up, make sure your right foot stays on the floor so that your right leg is pulled along by the power of your hip flexors. You don't need to strain or do any work with the foot. Lower your right knee until your leg is long and your foot goes straight down to where it began.

Each time you slide your right knee up, lower your head and notice the big gap under your right elbow, between your right hand and your shoulder. Look down to see your knee coming up, as though you were curious to read some message written there. Indulging in your curiosity promotes brain growth. When your knee straightens, turn your head to the left to relieve your neck. Make several lazy movements that way. Remember that your left arm is down at your side, near your pelvis. Every so often, you may have to readjust the position of your right hand and shoulder.

6. Now lie on your back with your arms and legs long and take a full rest. Feel the difference between your two sides. Earlier in the lesson, I asked you to notice the contrast between your two shoulders and between your two hips. What is that contrast like now? Is part of you more expanded? Which side of your body feels younger? Now let's make the other side of your body feel younger.

7. Roll onto your stomach, put your right arm down near your hip, and turn your face to the left. Without moving, imagine the ideal place to stand your left hand. Remember, it's an experiment. Imagining will allow your brain to map out the coordinates of the movement. Once you have imagined it clearly, bend your left elbow and stand your left hand, with your legs a comfortable distance apart. Aim your fingers away from yourself to the left and spread them apart easily so that your hand feels wide. Make sure your elbow is in the air, pointing toward the ceiling. Before you begin moving, find a good distance between your left hand and shoulder so that, as your left shoulder blade pulls back over your rib cage toward your spine, you can get your elbow completely straight without having to move your hand. You will feel your ribs yielding as you feel your shoulder moving left and right.

Imagine the movement a few times and then practice pulling your shoulder blade back until your left elbow straightens. Make sure your hand doesn't move but stays in the spot you chose for it.

The next time you slide your shoulder blade back toward your spine and straighten your left elbow, keep your arm straight, easily rolling your pelvis right and left, and observe how your pelvis and your rib cage can move underneath your shoulder. Remember, in order for the shoulder blade to return, your elbow bends so that your hand does not need to move.

Leave this movement and rest your elbow on the floor.

8. Roll your pelvis to the right so that your left hip lifts off the floor. Feel the softness in the back of your left knee each time you roll. Don't draw your knee up yet. Just observe that the knee has a tendency to begin bending, that the beginning of pulling the knee up lies in the way you organize your back and pelvis.

Pause.

9. Now stand on your left hand, fingers facing left and elbow in the air. Find the most comfortable place where you can push the most with your hand if you need to. Roll your pelvis so that your left hip comes off the floor and slide the inside of your left knee up near your waist. Then slide it down, making sure your left foot stays on the floor. Do this several times.

10. As your left knee comes up, begin to bring your head down, as though to read a cryptic message on your left knee. Go slowly and without strain. When is it best for you to breathe out?

To relieve your neck, each time your leg straightens, turn your head to the right. Let the whole movement be lighter and easier each time, until it feels smooth enough to imagine that you are doing it with almost no friction, as though on ice or a sheet of glass covered with oil. How would you organize your body to make it that simple?

Leave this movement, roll over, and rest on your back with your arms and legs long. Observe whether new parts of yourself feel flatter on the floor or more expanded. Take a moment to feel what's changed in your body.

11. Roll onto your stomach with your legs comfortably apart. Stand both hands on the floor with both elbows pointing toward the ceiling and your fingers spread apart, facing away from yourself. Put your forehead on the floor. I call this the "Alligator" position.

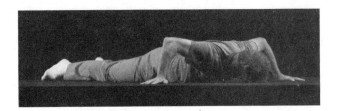

Draw your right knee and your head toward each other so that your head is looking underneath your right elbow at your knee. Then straighten the right knee as you draw the left knee and your head toward each other. Alternate this way a few times. Rest on your back with your arms and legs long. Observe the sensations in your chest, rib cage, and back.

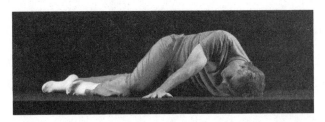

Roll onto your stomach into the Alligator position. Slide your right shoulder blade backward to straighten your right elbow as you roll your head to face right and draw your right knee up. As you straighten your right leg, simultaneously roll your head to face left and straighten your left elbow as you bring your left knee up. Pause and rest on your stomach in any way that is comfortable.

In this way, you can roll across your stomach and obtain maximum motion in your shoulder blades and spine.

Rest on your stomach with your head in its most comfortable position.

12. Return to the Alligator position. Slowly look up toward the ceiling and feel your back begin to extend as you straighten both elbows. Then come back down again. Look up and down several times, feeling the integration of the muscles of your pelvis and back with those of your shoulders and arms, so that nothing is working too hard.

As you look up, let your head and chest lift off the floor. Feel the parts of your body peeling off the floor in a neat sequence. Then put them down, part by part. Go up and down like this several times. Slowly lower yourself back to the floor. With your hands in a firm position, lift your head to look out beyond yourself and slowly draw your left knee up, as you did before. Can you look over your left shoulder to see your foot? Then slowly lower your left leg and look over your right shoulder as you draw up your right knee to see your right foot. Alternate drawing one knee up after the other as you turn your head to look over your shoulder toward your feet.

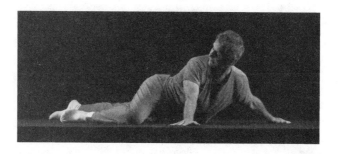

Change Your Age Tip: If you observe the constant rolling of your pelvis as your legs alternately slide up and down, you'll find that there's no strain in the movement. Don't feel compelled to look at your feet. If you can simply look behind yourself over each shoulder, you'll experience a renewed amount of movement in your neck, shoulders, and trunk from this lesson.

Rest for a few moments on your back and scan your body.

13. When you stand up, take a little time to notice whether you turn more easily and whether your chest feels more elevated. Do you feel wider? Is it easier to stand straight? How many years easier?

Lesson 18: ALTERNATE SIDE-SITTING OVER THE KNEES

● **Intention:** To learn how to organize yourself to go from side-sitting to a crawling position by using your forces against the ground, just as you did when you were very young.

● **Starting Position:** Take a side-sitting position on your left side, with your hands on the floor in front of you. If it is too difficult to side-sit on the left side, side-sit on the right for a moment.

In this movement, you want to minimize any frictional forces on the ground so that your knees don't get irritated. You can place a sheet over your pad or carpet to minimize the drag. Occasionally stop moving and imagine how you can reduce friction and make this movement lighter for yourself.

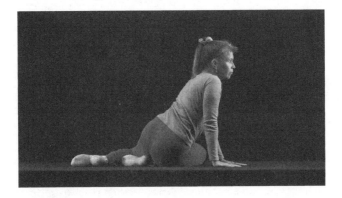

1. While pushing down on the floor with both hands, roll up over your left knee and bring your pelvis up until you are approximately on all fours.

2. Still pushing down on the floor with both hands, lift your pelvis up over your left knee and slide your left leg backward as you slide your right leg forward and sit on your right hip.

    Pause for a moment there on all fours.

3. Alternate the sliding of your legs and sit on your left hip. Sit from side to side this way a few times. This may be a familiar movement from early childhood.

    One reason for switching the legs forward and backward and lifting your pelvis up and down is to reduce friction. Reducing friction makes the movements of your lower extremities feel much lighter. Do this movement only a few times until it gets easier because you've reduced the friction.

    Then roll yourself up over both knees onto all fours again.

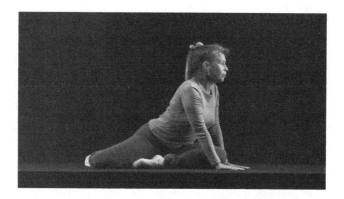

4. Stop on all fours and rest. Go back to the floor by bringing one knee forward and the other knee back while rolling softly onto your back. Rest with your arms and legs long and do a State of the Body Scan.

Lesson 19: FINDING THE TWO HALVES OF YOUR BODY

● **Intention:** To improve your balance by developing a stronger sense of the centerline of your body in relation to your limbs. You will learn to stabilize your hips and shoulders without stiffness.

● **Starting Position:** Start on your hands and knees. Balance on the floor so that your knees are not too close to your hands or too far away. Imagine a string dropping straight from your shoulder through your wrist and another string dropping straight from your hip through your knee, on both sides. Now your joints should be balanced and in alignment, and you are in a good crawling posture. Make sure your back is neither collapsed and sunken nor curved up toward the ceiling. Make sure your head is in a comfortable position.

Change Your Age Tip: If this position is too hard on your wrists, make fists so that you can rest your weight through the knuckles of your fists.

   If the floor bothers your knees, put some padding under them. A gardening pad is ideal; a folded towel may work even better.

1. Lift your left arm from the floor so that you feel your left shoulder rise toward the ceiling. Observe that the pressure into the floor increases under your right arm and your knees. Notice how your trunk rotates toward your left shoulder. Do this movement a few times, until you feel that your arm can dangle like a long piece of wet spaghetti even though your left shoulder is rising and your trunk is turning.

    Rest by sitting back on your heels, with your chest and head down on the floor. If that's not a comfortable resting position, then lie on your back.

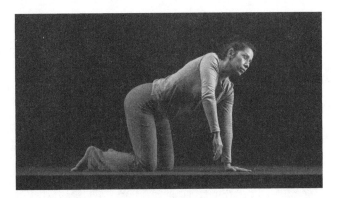

2. Once again, come to your balanced position on all fours and experiment with lifting your right arm the same way you lifted your left. Remember how useful it is to imagine a movement before performing it. Is it easier on this arm, or more difficult? Again, allow your trunk to move freely and feel your right shoulder rising toward the ceiling as your arm dangles.

Change Your Age Tip: Many people cannot feel the difference between the movement of their shoulder and trunk and the possibility of independent motion of their arm. This is why many people can't turn their head easily when they swim and why many golfers injure their necks on their follow-through. The movements in this lesson will develop independence and greater freedom of motion in your arm because you won't be engaging all the muscles in your head, neck, and shoulders when you engage your arm.

Rest as before.

3. Return to the crawling position. Now can you lift the right side of your pelvis and your right hip toward the ceiling and let your right knee and leg dangle?

   Make sure that your right foot stays resting on the floor and that the muscles on the side of the lifting right leg don't pull that leg out to the side. In this way, you'll feel the muscles in your back and the forces you use against the ground with your hands and your other leg helping you lift your right leg.

   Rest so that you take the weight off your wrists.

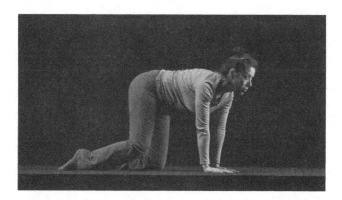

4. Return to the crawling position and do the same movement on the other side so that your left knee and leg can move up and down without using any muscles in the leg itself. Can you feel how your trunk organizes and mobilizes your limbs into motion?

   Rest so that you take the weight off your wrists.

5. Now simultaneously lift your right shoulder and your right hip toward the ceiling. Make sure both your right arm and leg are dangling as you balance on your other hand and knee. If you can, turn your head to look over your right shoulder toward the ceiling and then down at your standing hand. This will build a lot of stability in the core muscles of your hips and shoulders and significantly improve your balance as well as the balance and strength of those joints.

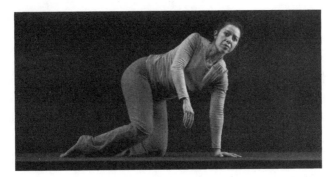

Rest on your back with your arms and legs long and notice whether you feel differences in the two sides of your body. Does one side feel more stable or stronger?

6. When you are ready, return to a crawling position and repeat Step 5 on the other side. Rest again on your back to finish. When you are ready, come to standing and observe how your body balances as you walk. Notice whether you feel more stable as you stand and walk.

Lesson 20: CRAWLING WITH YOUR KNEES UP AND DOWN

● **Intention:** To rapidly adjust from your hands and knees to bringing your feet under yourself. You will regain years of flexibility in your hips and lower back.

● **Starting Position:** Start on your hands and knees, as in the previous lesson.

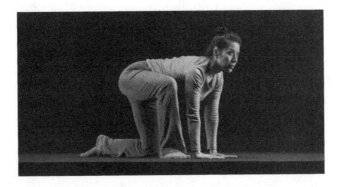

1. Bring your right leg forward so that you can stand your right foot somewhere on the floor. Do this several times and experiment with

different places where you can solidly stand your foot. You might be able to stand your foot near your right arm.

Change Your Age Tip: If you stand on your fists, you'll find that it's easier to move your hip and your leg. You might also discover a feeling of more space.

Rest on your back, with your arms and legs long, and observe the feeling of your right leg. How is it different from the left? Which leg is younger?

2. Return to the crawling position and explore standing on your left foot in different places. You might stand it wide, away from your body, or close in, under the middle of your body. Find where it is most solid.

Change Your Age Tip: There is no good movement without breathing, so let your breath be part of the movement of your legs. Observe what you do with your head and neck that might make the movement easier for you—for example, you can look at your foot as you stand on it and look out and away when you return to both knees.

Rest on your back, with your arms and legs long, and feel your contact with the floor.

Advanced Variation on Lesson 20:
CRAWLING WITH KNEES UP AND DOWN

● **Intention:** To increase your agility in moving from the floor to a standing position. You'll also develop deep muscles in your trunk and back as well as your hips and shoulders that will keep you agile and quick.

I use this movement with hundreds of people in back care programs and core-strengthening programs. It's been found to be extremely effective. It may be difficult at first, but it's worth trying. This is actually a very efficient way to have both feet stand under the pelvis, and it can be the fastest and easiest way to rise from the floor.

● **Starting Position:** Return to all fours and recheck your balance and alignment.

1. Lift both of your arms off the floor until you are upright on both knees. Then return your hands to the floor slowly. Do this movement several times.

    Rest on your back.

2. Return to the crawling position. The next movement is one that you can show off at barbecues or cocktail parties to impress your friends with your newfound youthful movement. Lift both of your knees off the floor and "jump" with your hands remaining on the floor until both feet are in a standing position.

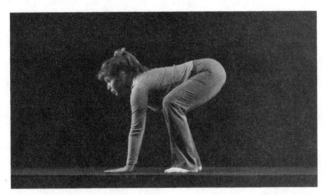

Then, in one movement, return your feet in preparation for softly landing on your knees and returning to a crawling position.

The next time you jump your feet into the air, land directly on both feet.

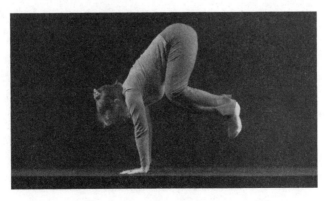

3. Once both feet are under you, it may be easy to let your hands lift off the floor as you move your pelvis forward and find yourself standing. Can you slowly go down, with your hands returning to the floor, and go back to the crawling position? Repeat these movements a few times until they become intuitive.

Rest on your back, with your arms and legs long, and feel the years peel away.

Lesson 21: UPRIGHT KNEELING

● **Intention:** To practice pelvic movements in order to reduce stress on your knees. Many people move their hips only from the hip joint and don't allow their pelvis and spine to be integrated into the action. This can put tremendous stress on your knees because you are using primarily the quadriceps muscle in your thigh. By practicing this movement, you can learn to allow your entire pelvis to move with your leg.

● **Starting Position:** Start this movement upright, on your knees, with your ankles pulled back so that you can push through your toes. Use a folded towel under your knees if needed.

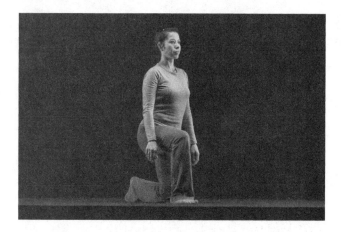

1. Bring your right leg forward and stand on your right foot. Then bring your right leg back and return to both knees. Do the same thing with

your left leg. Now alternate standing on your right foot and your left foot a few times. Which side is easier? The movement of your pelvis as you lift your leg is the same movement you use to climb stairs. Observe how much you need to move your pelvis and trunk to complete the action of bringing your leg forward to stand on one foot. Feel your pelvis move.

Rest lying on your back with your arms and legs long for a few moments.

2. Return to both knees, with both your ankles and toes bent. Without using your arms to assist yourself, step your right foot forward again, as before. While pushing down through your right foot—as well as the toes on your left foot—come to standing. Use the same right leg to return to the floor position where you began.

3. Repeat the same action leading with your left foot and leg.

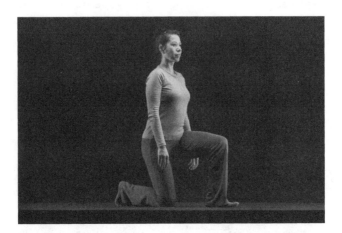

Which side is easier for you? It could be that the side on which it's easier to move from upright kneeling to standing on the foot is not necessarily the side on which it's easier to push through one leg to standing. The ability to come to standing through one leg is one of the more difficult challenges we face as we age.

Change Your Age Tip: Do not repeat this lesson if it irritates your knees or your hips. You can do the lesson near a substantial piece of furniture for support until it becomes easier to do without such support or without using your arms.

POSITION 4: CROUCHING

We may use other positions to learn movement, but in crouching we really learn to move.

Crouching involves the most direct interaction between the largest muscles in your body and gravity. It's something that only mammals perform and that humans use all the time on their way to standing or sitting. We pass from the horizontal to the vertical line through crouching. Crouching deserves extensive attention because many people, as they get older, either lose their ability to crouch or are pulled into an immobilizing crouch by pain and stiffness. Most people who want to move better go down into a crouching position because they want to spring forward, up, or to the side. In activities from tennis to gardening, we crouch in order to increase our ability to perform the task in front of us.

The other aspect of crouching—resting—is actually the opposite of movement. Think of baseball players on the field or basketball players on the court with their hands resting on their thighs. The back relaxes, the neck can relax, and the flexors can let go. When you practice crouching, you can breathe much more deeply. Your body can experience another kind of balance between its front and back.

Crouching can take us to squatting, which lengthens all the major muscle groups that we are intent on stretching. To learn to move deeper into and out of a squat ensures a more flexible body. Crouching can also lead us to actions like standing and jumping. For example, if you imagine jumping a small amount over a thin line on the floor, your body will organize its parts in such a way that would prepare you for easier standing and automatically lengthen you from crouching to standing.

Lesson 22: THROUGH CROUCHING TO STANDING

● **Intention:** To help you become more agile while moving up and down and discover that your legs can be strong in many different ways, depending on which muscles you recruit and the angle at which you move.

● **Starting Position:** Roll onto your hands and knees, as in Lesson 20. Settle comfortably and feel that you are rested on your hands and knees. If your wrists bother you, rest on your fists.

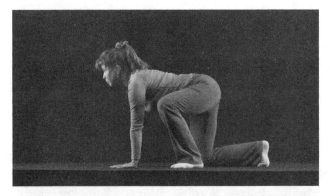

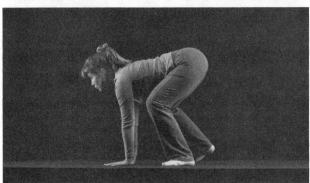

1. Bring your left leg forward and stand your left foot on the floor. Now push through your left foot and stand your right foot on the floor.

   Slowly lift your head to look at the horizon and stand up. Keep your head up while you look around with curiosity.

2. Bend down by moving your pelvis backward and bending your knees a little, until your hands touch the floor.

3. Once your hands touch the floor, can you step back with the foot that's easiest for you? Step back and set that knee on the floor. Then step back with the other foot and set that knee on the floor.

4. Come back up again systematically, setting your favorite foot forward, the one that is easier for you. Then set the other foot forward. Feel that you have some weight on both your hands and your feet.

Lift your head to look at the horizon and stand up.

Change Your Age Tip: You most likely tend to lead with the same foot most, if not all, of the time. Each time you go up and down, change the foot that leads. Alternating this way, you may find that the going gets easier with the less familiar foot.

Even people with knee problems find that they can do this, as long as they don't do it on a hard surface.

● ● ● **Body Intelligence Reminder for Advanced Variation on Lesson 22:** In some lessons, you might have difficulty because your brain and your body are not familiar with the movements, or perhaps the movements are ones you have forgotten how to do. Eventually, you will gain the body awareness to practice the lessons well.

Advanced Variation on Lesson 22:
THROUGH CROUCHING TO STANDING

● **Intention:** To improve your dexterity while maneuvering between bending positions, crouching positions, and standing positions.

You will feel stronger and lighter if you do these movements every day. People who have had hip joint surgery or knee replacement surgery can safely do these movements.

● **Starting Position:** Start in a standing position with your legs shoulder width apart. If your legs are too close together, this movement can strain your back. Make sure you are looking out and breathing easily.

1. Place your hands on the floor while still looking out. Then simply hop your feet backward and put your knees down on the floor.

   When you hop back, hop far enough to make enough space by your arms for your knees to touch the floor.

2. Imagine lifting your knees up and hopping forward toward your hands. After *imagining* this backward-and-forward jumping movement, perform it two or three times.

3. Look out and stand up by pushing your pelvis forward as your arms and head rise and you straighten your knees.

   Think of your pelvis going forward each time you stand up, and you'll find the movement to be less work, less effortful, than if you think of lifting your weight up.

4. Go down and place your hands on the floor again. Simply hop backward to return to your knees and hop forward a few times until you feel the easiest place to return to crouching and standing. When you get a sense of this movement, you can simply lift your knees and hop forward in one movement, as you would do if you were catching a wave and mounting your surfboard.

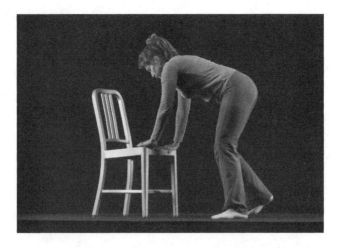

Change Your Age Tip: Another variation on the movement of standing up from the floor is to use furniture, as we explored in Lesson 15. You can use a table, a chair, a sofa, a counter—almost anything. As long as you can get up to your knees and your hands can push down on whatever furniture you are using, you can step up and down with one foot after the other and move your pelvis forward.

Sometimes people get up using furniture that is so directly in front of them that they can't move their pelvis forward. Be sure to allow enough room around yourself to do this movement.

Lesson 23: HOW TO APPROACH SQUATTING

● **Intention:** To discover that you can squat again. It's easier to learn to squat because squatting the right way is less stressful on the joints and muscles. Mastering squatting makes it easier to crouch properly. You will find it easier to retain the ability to squat if you can move up and down from crouching to squatting. Remember, *reversible* movement from one position to another will always help you retain an ability—more than simply practicing getting into difficult positions.

This short lesson requires that you move your back and spine in new and perhaps unusual ways. This is necessary to lift the knees from the floor to squatting and then return them to the floor.

● **Starting Position:** Start in a crouching position. Bend your knees enough so that you can rest your hands on your thighs near your knees. Align yourself so that you can rest into your arms and shoulders. Feel that you are free to look around and that you are relaxed enough to breathe easily. Think of how you might feel if you were watching a sporting event and had decided to stand in a relaxed, but alert manner. Remember, crouching is a position of both relaxation and readiness.

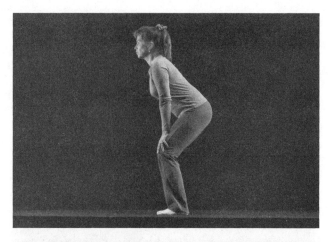

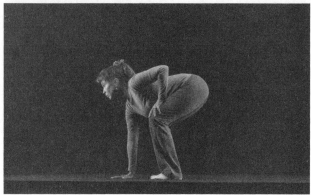

1. Reach with your right hand down to the floor in front of yourself. Keep your left hand on your knee. Return to the crouching position. Try this movement of putting your hand down to the floor and returning it to your knee a few times on each side until you've determined which side is easier. Rest in the crouching position.

2. Now place both hands on the floor. Slowly bend your knees until they come close to the floor, and then return to a squatting position by lifting your knees from the floor. Do this several times until you discover where you can put your hands so that your knees land on the floor very close to your hands. Ideally, your hands will be very close to your knees.

   Rest in standing.

3. Return to the crouching position. Let your hands go to the floor first, and then lower your pelvis until you are in a squatting position. Keep your hands on the floor. (If your heels are not able to touch the floor, you are still in a squatting position.)

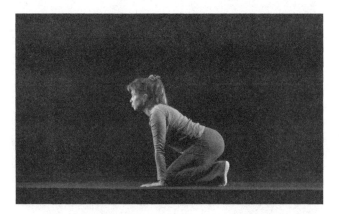

Move your knees forward to touch the floor and then backward until you find yourself squatting again. Do this a few times and adjust where you put your hands until the squatting becomes easier. You will find yourself rocking over the balls of your feet. Some people can get their heels down, but others can't; it makes no difference as long as you feel your knees going up and down behind your arms and your feet rocking.

Then, as you lift your pelvis in the air, lift your hands from the floor and return to a crouching position.

Rest in standing by walking around a bit. Observe if your walking feels easier.

Lesson 24: CROUCHING FOR YOUR LIFE

● **Intention:** To improve your speed of motion and significantly help your balance. In many sports, the speed with which a player moves from a crouch into action is important. In this lesson, it's also important to return to crouching in a relaxed, alert manner. Play with this quick sideways movement until you feel you can cross your legs and move quickly to either side.

● **Starting Position:** Start in the crouching position, as in the previous lesson. Re-member to bend your knees enough to enable you to place your hands on your thighs near your knees, as if you were resting from a standing position—or as if you were an outfielder waiting for the ball to go into play, or a basketball player waiting for a time-out to end.

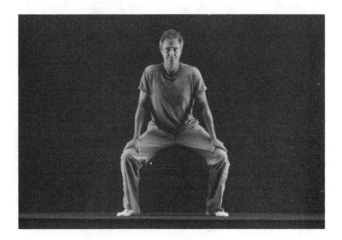

1. From this relaxed crouch, move your right foot in front of yourself and to the left side of your body, beyond your left foot. Your arms might have to be free. Return immediately to a relaxed, crouched position. Do this several times, until you can make the movement quickly and smoothly, as if you were dancing.

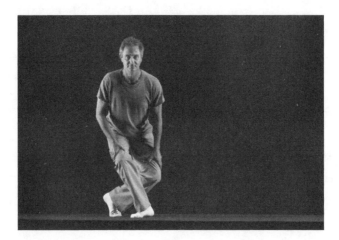

2. Do the same thing on the other side so that your left foot goes to the right side of your body, beyond your right foot. Return to a crouching position. Repeat several times and explore which side is easier.

3. Once you've mastered going to each side, move side to side the same way. Return to a crouch, and this time take each foot in back of the other one as you cross to the other side of the body.

Walk around and feel if you are more alert and ready.

POSITION 5: STANDING AND WALKING

It sounds obvious, but it's not. People stand for a reason. We stand as we wait in line at the supermarket, subway, or bus stop. We stand to stretch after sitting. We stand as preparation for walking or going for a run. How we stand is influenced by our purpose. In standing there's an implied orientation to the outer world. Practicing the simple acts of standing from sitting, walking with different intentions, and standing with different amounts of effort and intensity can create an immediate sense of joy.

Also, to many people walking is the most enjoyable form of exercise. Not to mention the fact that it is essential for getting people from place to place. Most people don't walk well, however, and are not even aware of the fact that they don't walk well. Many people simply don't enjoy walking, or they find it unpleasant when they have to speed up. Sometimes people don't like to walk because their balance isn't very good or because walking makes their hips or knees ache or feel stiff.

In this section, you will learn how to find much better balance than you've ever known before, and you will experience much smoother movement in your hips, knees, ankles, and feet. Not only will these lessons save the feet and knees of walkers from stress, but they are also very good lessons for runners. Finally, what you learn here will give you a more elegant and graceful walk, which will enable you to more fully enjoy one of life's major activities. You will have more spring in your step and a more youthful bounce in your walk.

Lesson 25: FREEING STIFF HIPS AND KNEES

● **Intention:** To create a more integrated relationship between your hips, ankles, and knees for greater mobility and balance. The relationship of hips to ankles and knees is poorly understood by most people. Sometimes a limitation in one of these joints inhibits the movement of the other two joints. Ideally, all three move together and, if one is limited, the other two simply move a little more. This is an excellent lesson as a tune-up for running or a slow walk in high heels.

● **Starting Position:** You will need to have a chair with a high enough back to enable you to stand next to it and comfortably place your fingers or hand on it without having to reach down or bend over.

1. Face the back of the chair and stand off to the left side so that you have room in front of you, with your right hand on the back of the chair. Bend your right knee just enough to lift your right heel off the floor. Repeat the motion several times. Do not lean more heavily on your hand.
2. Now lift the ball of your foot from the floor so that all the weight rocks back to the right heel. Your left leg remains stable. Check that you can breathe and do the motion at the same time.

Change Your Age Tip: When your right heel comes off the floor, can you feel your right knee moving forward lightly and your hip softly folding? To lift the ball of your foot, feel what's necessary to do on your stable left leg and with your back and pelvis. Be sure to keep your upper body easily upright so that you can look out and around.

---

3. Now rock back and forth from the heel of your right foot to the ball of that foot. You do not need to move your whole body forward and backward, but you might find your right hip moving forward and backward slightly. Be sure not to exert pressure on the chair.

    Walk around for a moment and notice any differences in your legs and feet while walking.

4. Return to your chair and place your left hand on the back while you stand to the right of the chair. As you did on the right side, first lift your left heel off the floor and observe how you do it lightly and easily. Can you feel the work of stabilizing yourself in the right hip?

5. Now lift the ball of your left foot from the floor. It might be easier or harder than when you did it on the right side.

6. Now rock from the ball to the heel of your left foot, making sure that your upper body feels free and your eyes can look up and out. Every so often, close your eyes to deepen the feeling and then open them to link the feeling with looking out. Rest by walking and feel what's happened to the motion of your legs and to your balance.

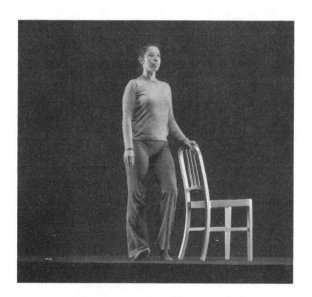

7. Return to the right side of your chair, with your left hand supporting yourself on the back of it. Alternately lift the ball of one foot and the heel of the other. So, for example, as the ball of your right foot lifts from the floor and you press on your right heel, your left heel picks up as you stand on the ball of your left foot. Make this a smooth and steady alternation. Do the movement very slowly at first and then learn to go quickly. Master all speeds.

Change Your Age Tip: Can you do this movement with your eyes closed, making sure that you're balanced and breathing and not gripping your chair? Then can you do it with your eyes open and looking to each side? Looking at the ceiling? While focusing on something in the room or out the window? Can you keep the movement going steadily whether your eyes are open or closed? If you feel safe enough, take your hand away from the back of the chair.

You will probably feel your hips shifting from side to side. Let that happen.

Rest and enjoy your new ability to walk more easily. See if your legs feel lighter and younger than before.

Lesson 26: IMPROVING BALANCE

● **Intention:** To greatly improve your balance and contribute to your enjoyment of walking.

Many people don't even realize that they have difficulties balancing because they have never been diagnosed with a balance disorder. However, a startling number of people avoid situations where their balance could be challenged, and these people frequently find themselves looking down at the floor or sidewalk whenever they move about.

● **Starting Position:** Stand with your feet shoulder width apart.

This lesson will be much easier to perform if you are standing next to a chair or at a wall or counter that you can touch to provide support. This lesson will challenge your balance, so make sure you feel comfortable and safe.

1. Cross your right leg over your left leg so that your ankles are crossed and your right foot is standing on the floor just outside your left foot. Make sure that your whole foot is on the floor and that both heels are down.

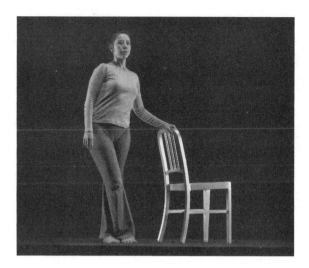

2. Slowly shift your hips left and right as far as it is comfortable to go. Reduce the effort you make to maintain balance. Do this enough times that you learn to feel secure and comfortable. Relax your jaw and look out into the room, breathing fully. Uncross your legs and rest while standing.

Change Your Age Tip: As you shift your hips, you will feel yourself pressing more on one foot and then the other. As your hips move from side to side, your head remains stationary.

---

3. Now cross your left foot in front of your right foot, so that your left foot is standing on the floor just outside your right foot. Again, oscillate your hips from side to side until you feel certain of how to organize your back, hips, head, neck, and shoulders, repeating until this feels like a natural movement. Uncross your legs and rest while standing.

4. Cross your right foot over your left foot again, as in Step 1. Now shift your head and shoulders from side to side. What do your hips need to do? Learn to make your body comfortable by using all of its parts. Gauge your comfort by the ease of your breathing. Uncross your legs and rest in standing.

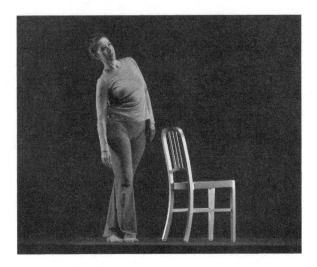

5. Cross your left foot over your right foot. Again, move your head and shoulders from side to side. Is it easier or harder with your legs crossed in this arrangement? Uncross your legs and rest while standing. After you have rested, walk around the room. Are you more aware of your hips?

6. Return to the chair or wall for some support. Once again, cross your right foot over your left foot so that your ankles are crossed and your right foot is standing outside your left foot. This time, move your pelvis forward and backward so that you press toward the balls of your feet and then toward your heels. If you are comfortable enough with this movement, you might be able to lift both heels off the floor when you go forward with your pelvis, and perhaps you can lift your toes and the balls of your feet when you push your pelvis backward. Uncross your legs and rest while standing.

Change Your Age Tip: As you move your pelvis forward and backward, let your arms, shoulders, and neck relax completely so that you can feel your head and your arms moving in opposition to your pelvis to help you balance. Your head will feel as if it's reaching forward and pulling backward.

---

7. Cross your left foot over your right foot so that your ankles are crossed with the left foot just outside the right foot. Oscillate your pelvis for-

ward and back, as in Step 6. Uncross your legs, rest, and then go for a short walk around the room.

8. Place one of your hands on the back of your chair or on the wall and again cross your right leg over your left leg. Stand tall, but comfortably. Turn your head to look around the room. As you do, look in back of yourself as far as possible. Look at the ceiling and the floor. Can you feel the adjustments that your hips need to make?

9. Recross your legs with the left one crossed in front. Continue looking around the room in this arrangement. Which way of crossing your legs gives you better balance? Take time to discover the answer for yourself. Rest in standing.

10. Stand with your right leg crossed over your left leg. Can you make a circle of pressure on the bottoms of your feet? Move your pelvis in a circle so that you feel as if both your pelvis and the bottoms of your feet are tracing circles, one in the air and one on the floor. Uncross your legs and rest in standing.

11. Cross your left leg over the right one and explore your circle of pressure this way. Which side creates the roundest, smoothest circles on the bottoms of your feet?

Rest by walking around the room. You might find that your legs can walk in a narrower path than usual.

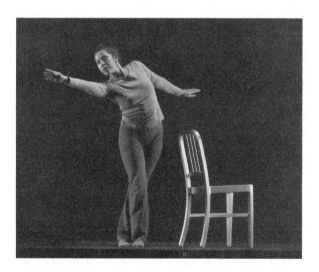

12. Once again cross your right leg over the left one and raise both of your arms out to your sides at the height of your shoulders. While you imagine holding on to two swords, lunge first to one side and then to the other, as far as you can reach, keeping your legs crossed. Can you also reach one arm in front of you and the other in back of you and alternate reaching forward and backward with your arms?

13. Try the same lunging and reaching actions of your arm in as many directions as possible with your left leg crossed over your right leg.

   Rest by going for a walk and notice if you can feel an improvement in your balance and a keener awareness of what you need to do with your hips to help yourself balance more easily. This will improve your balance in all situations, including walking in narrow high heels.

Lesson 27: THE ULTIMATE WALKING LESSON

● **Intention:** To learn how to move your legs more easily by using your arms and shoulders. When we walk, our shoulders and hips need to move in opposition to each other, as do our elbows and knees and our hands and feet. The more we reduce this counter-rotation of the upper and lower body, the stiffer and more awkward our way of walking becomes. The more we *increase* this counter-rotation, the faster our hips and legs can move.

● **Starting Position:** Stand with your feet a comfortable distance apart.

1. Slowly and carefully turn your chest and shoulders from side to side without moving your pelvis at all. You might need to look at a mirror to make sure you are really able to do this. Do not make the movement large; instead, work to make it distinct and clearly felt.

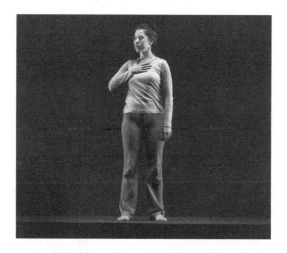

2. Now turn your pelvis from side to side, keeping your chest and shoulders stationary. Again, focus your attention on the clarity and simplicity of the movement; the size of the movement is unimportant. Rest in standing.

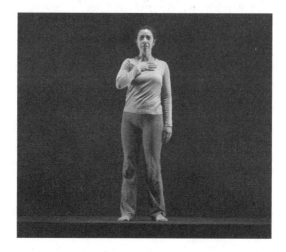

3. Stand comfortably with your feet apart, as you would have them in preparation to walk. Bend your elbows until your forearms are parallel to the floor, and make fists with your hands. Soften your knees so that they are not locked straight and slide your right fist forward as you take your left elbow backward. Then alternate so that your left fist pushes forward and your right elbow pulls backward. Alternate many times.

Change Your Age Tip: As you move your arms, pump them forward and backward. Let them swing freely so that your shoulders move forward and backward and you feel your chest turning from side to side. As you do this, can you feel the result in your pelvis? Is it stable, or can you allow it to move slightly so that it turns in the opposite direction of your shoulders and chest? Let the swinging of your arms become larger until you feel the effect on your waist and pelvis.

Rest while standing or walking.

4. Now place your right hand on the side of your right thigh near the hip, keeping your elbow straight. Do the same with your left hand on your left thigh. Go for a walk in which your arms weld your hips and shoulders together, eliminating any and all counter-rotation in your body.

5. Can you walk with your right hand on your right thigh and your left arm swinging freely? Since most people move one arm and shoulder more than the other, you may be exaggerating a habit you already have.

   Be sure that you feel how the right hip and right shoulder move forward at the same time.

   Release the right hand and walk normally.

6. Put your left hand against your thigh and move your hip and shoulder together on this side. It might feel either more awkward or more coordinated than the other side. Release your left hand and walk normally.

7. Walk as you exaggerate the forward-and-backward movement of your shoulders. Try to keep your head more or less centered as you do this, and allow your arms a larger amplitude. Notice the effect this has on your hips and legs.

8. Now exaggerate the motion of your pelvis as it turns forward to follow each leg. You might feel your shoulders still moving in the exaggerated manner.

9. Sense the motion of your knees as you walk and exaggerate the forward movement as you walk. Think of aiming your knees toward someplace you want to reach and let your knees reach for that place as you go.

10. Walk normally for a while and observe whether you have more awareness of how your trunk, shoulders, and legs work in harmony when you walk. As you're walking, play with exaggerating your arm swing

for a while, then your shoulder movement. Occasionally exaggerate your hip rotation for a bit, then the forward-reaching motion of your knees. As you experiment with all these possibilities, you'll notice that your walk has become more graceful because you have so many body parts in motion.

Change Your Age Tip: As with the previous lesson, the more parts of your body you move as you walk, the more graceful your walk will be. The fewer parts of your body you move in response to the other parts when you walk, the more effort, resistance, and awkwardness will appear in your walk. When you first move many parts of your body fully as you walk, it may feel exaggerated. But don't worry—nobody will notice. And if they do, all they'll see is that you look more elegant and graceful.

Advanced Variation on Lesson 27:
THE ULTIMATE WALKING LESSON— CONTINUATION FOR RUNNING

● **Intention:** To give you that burst of speed you need when dashing across the street in traffic.

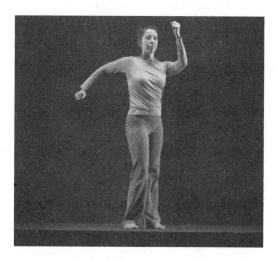

Following all the steps in Lesson 27, continue doing Step 10 with a larger arm swing until you feel how your arms can pump your pelvis and legs, as if you were running by using your upper body. Many people don't realize that this is the secret of track-and-field athletes: They use their arms to move their legs more easily and faster.

Lesson 28: STANDING ON THE HIGHEST POINT OF THE HIP

● **Intention:** To find the highest point of your hip joint so that you can include a feeling for this point in your way of standing and walking. Everyone who has any concern about their hip joint as they age should do this lesson.

Many arthritic and osteoporotic conditions are aggravated and accelerated when weight from the pelvis to the head of the femur (or thigh bone) does not go in the direction best aligned to maintain the strength of the bones and the joint. In the ball-and-socket joint of your hip, where you bear weight determines how the internal structure of the femur grows and changes over time.

The best place to bear weight is at the highest point of the hip joint, but many people have the habit of sinking in their hips or standing so that the weight of the pelvis is lower on the ball-and-socket joint of the hip.

● **Starting Position:** Stand with your feet as wide as your hips. You might feel comfortable doing this near a piece of furniture or a wall to help give you balance and support if you need it. Imagine that half of your body is one piece, one unit, from your left leg and your left foot all the way through your spine and torso to the top of your head; think of those parts of your body as containing an unbendable stick. You can only move at your right hip joint.

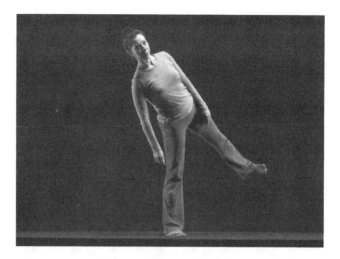

1. Bear more weight on your right leg so that you can lift your left foot and leg out to the left side of your body. Your head will have to move exactly the same amount to the right. Then return to standing on both feet. Let your arms hang freely and do the movement slowly several times.

Change Your Age Tip: Be very careful not to tilt your neck to the right, or your chest or any part of your spine; be sure to stay on top of your right hip joint. You will be moving your pelvis on top of your hip joint. There is no need to lift your left leg very far.

---

2. Stop and go for a walk. Do you feel the difference in your hips and legs? How do they support you differently?

3. Imagine the same movement on your right side: Your body doesn't bend except at your left hip as your right foot and leg lift off the floor to the right side and your head moves equally to the left. Now you will be balancing on top of your left hip joint. Don't try to go too far. Go as slowly as you can. Feel that your right foot and leg move exactly the same distance to the right that your head moves to the left. Make sure your trunk is truly unbendable.

   You may want to go back and practice again on the other side. Observe which side is easier.

4. Stop and go for a walk. Feel how your pelvis sits high on your hip joints. If you feel fatigued in the muscles around your hip joints, lie down and rest for a moment before continuing.

Change Your Age Tip: As you do these movements, all of the stabilizing muscles of your hip joints awaken and, for some people, become fully activated for the first time. The secret is in going slowly and carefully to keep everything immobile except the movement over the hip joint.

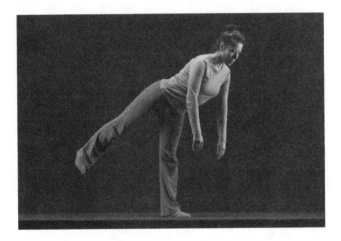

5. Return to standing. Now imagine again that the right side of your body is an unbendable unit. As you bring your right foot forward, your head will go back exactly the same distance. Take your foot and leg backward and let your head go forward the exact same distance. Do this several times. Be sure you are not arching your back and that all movement is directly over the right hip joint.

    Rest. Go for a walk. Observe any changes you feel in your head and hips and how your pelvis sits above your legs.

6. Repeat the same movement on the other side. As you go back and forth over your right hip joint, relax your shoulders and let your arms hang freely in front or in back of yourself, wherever they want to go.

Pause. Observe how you are standing. Feel whether you are higher above your legs. Go for a walk and observe what's new compared to your usual way of walking. Can you sense your hip joints and the muscles around them in a new way? Practicing this lesson every day will give you better balance and stronger, more stable hips.

● ***Body Intelligence Reminder for Lessons 29 and 30:*** You might want to rest on your back with your arms and legs long and do a brief State of the Body Scan before continuing with the next two lessons.

Before you start jumping or hopping, make sure you can bounce up and down on your heels a few times. Bounce on your heels until you feel how to make the movement smooth so it doesn't disturb your equilibrium.

Recent research has shown that jumping and hopping are the best activities for building stronger bones and preventing osteoporosis. Practice the next two lessons for short periods of time but at frequent intervals.

Lesson 29: JUMPING TO DISCOVER YOUR POSTURE

● **Intention:** To use jumping to help you rethink your relationship to your posture. Most of the time we think of posture in a very abstract way; in reality, our posture changes depending on the movement we are going to do next. Good posture for jumping is different from good posture for standing and looking up at the stars or from the posture you might take to talk with a friend.

If you were to make very small jumps with your toes still on the ground, you would find yourself—in your hips and knees—getting stronger each day. It's unimportant how high you jump; what's important is how you land. Always land in a posture from which you are prepared to jump again a few times.

● **Starting Position:** Stand as if you had a piece of tape on the floor in front of your feet. As you stand, imagine that you are going to jump just beyond that tape. With your posture, you will be preparing yourself to jump forward a small distance, and that preparation embodies a kind of postural ideal. As soon as we even think about jumping over a tape on the floor, most of us improve our posture: We bring our pelvis slightly backward, open our chest, and move into a better skeletal alignment. If you lean too far backward or are too slumped in your chest, you will find it difficult to look ahead and jump forward even a little bit.

1. Don't jump first, but think: Where will I put my feet over the tape?
   The first place you're going to jump is forward, and the elevation should be minimal. Imagine how you are going to jump forward. How must you prepare yourself for that movement?
   Jump forward two or three times.
2. Now prepare yourself to jump backward and do so two or three times. Jump forward and backward a few times, breathing easily with a relaxed jaw.

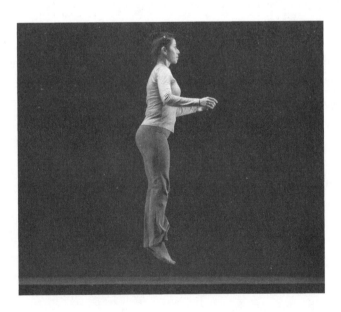

3. Jump to the right side twice. Then jump to the left side twice. Can you jump forward, again just a small distance?

   Pause. Remember how your organize your body diffeerently for each direction you jump.

4. Jump up a small distance and, as you do, turn 90 degrees to your right when you land. Jump again while turning 90 degrees to your left. Again jump 90 degrees to your left. And then 90 degrees to the right so that you are back where you started.

Change Your Age Tip: Jumping is an excellent practice for postural control, balance, bone building, and joint strengthening. The trick to useful jumping is to not jump too high, so there is no shock to your body. Another trick is to do something besides simply jump—like turning your body, which improves your vestibular system (the balancing mechanism in your inner ear).

---

5. Breathe easily and make sure you can turn your head easily. Let your body feel soft. Now perform three jumps forward. Make them small, coordinated jumps, not too high and not too far. Rest by walking or lying on the floor.

Body Intelligence Reminder for Advanced Variation on Lesson 29:
Again, don't compete with yourself to do an advanced variation before you are ready.

Advanced Variation on Lesson 29:
JUMPING TO DISCOVER YOUR POSTURE

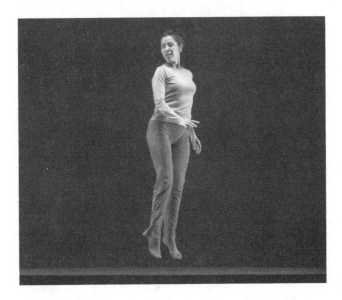

Can you jump to your right 180 degrees to face behind yourself? Recover your balance and inner equilibrium. Then jump to the right to face behind yourself again. Now jump to the left 180 degrees. And then 180 degrees again to return to where you started.

Rest while standing.

Change Your Age Tip: One way to evaluate your capacities is to see how far away you are from being able to jump and turn 360 degrees in either direction and land with complete stability. Even some skilled athletes and dancers can't maintain equilibrium when they first try it. On the other hand, people who feel far from being able to jump can develop this ability gradually by practicing as many lessons as they can in this program.

Lesson 30: HOPPING FOR HEALTH

● **Intention:** To help you maintain the coordination of your ankles, knees, hips, and back in order to improve your ability to climb stairs, run, and jump. This is also a great bone-building exercise that stretches your brain as it improves your coordination. The leg we feel more secure hopping on is the leg we tend to favor in our balance, walking, and running. If you are running fast and have to jump over a puddle of water or a small creek, your brain automatically knows which leg you will lead with and land on. In research, the favored side has been shown to be invariable, and in fact, people can feel quite uncomfortable if they lead with and land on their less favored leg.

This hopping lesson can change fundamental habits that you have had all of your life by teaching you to divide the work of your legs more evenly.

● **Starting Position:** Stand with your feet a comfortable distance apart.

1. Shift your pelvis to the left until all of your weight is on your left leg. Bend your right leg and raise it so that you bounce your left heel on the floor. You will have to raise yourself onto the ball of your left foot to do this. Do this movement a few times until it feels easy to bounce your heel on the floor. Hit the floor firmly with your heel.
   Pause.
2. Shift your pelvis to the right and practice the same action, now bouncing your right heel. Observe whether it is easier to do this movement on the left side or the right side. Practice until you know.
   Rest and walk around the room.
3. Shift your pelvis once again to the left side and make the action described in Step 1 larger, until you are hopping on your left leg. Don't make a large hop, but feel that you can leave the floor completely and safely land. A smaller hop will be more beneficial in this lesson than a high hop.
   Pause.

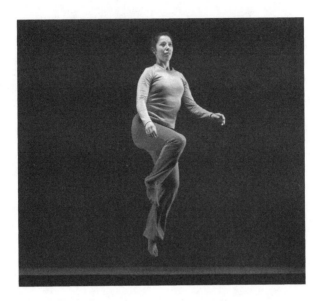

4. Hop on your right leg and observe whether it is easier.

5. Now hop several times on your left leg as you slowly turn in a complete circle to the left. Maintain your body awareness so that you can do this action with a relaxed jaw and soft breathing. Stop if this action makes you dizzy.

   Pause. Catch your breath and regain your equilibrium.

   Now hop on your left leg, turning to the right. Which direction is easier?

6. Shift your weight to your right leg and hop several times on that leg to turn in a complete circle to the right.

   Rest for a moment. Use your mind to relax any stress you might have accumulated in your back, shoulders, jaw, or belly.

7. Hop on your right foot again in a circle going to the left.

   Rest in standing, then stroll around the room and observe how you feel. How many years has it been since you jumped and hopped this frequently? A little bit every day is the fastest way to strengthen bones and many muscle groups and regain more youthful movement.

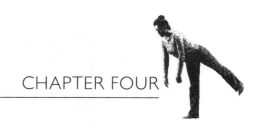

CHAPTER FOUR

YOUR BODY, YOUR TIME

Customizing the Program to Fit Your Individual Needs

CONGRATULATIONS! You have completed all 30 lessons. You may not always have time to do all of the lessons at once, in sequence, and you don't always have to. You may have favorite lessons that you want to repeat every day, perhaps as something new to add to your current fitness program. Sometimes you might want to stay on the floor, and on other days you might want to work with the lessons sitting in a chair. You will have different reasons for doing these lessons at different times—for example, to energize yourself in the morning, to relax yourself in the evening, or to give yourself an afternoon movement break from work. Here are some ideas on how you can customize a sequence of lessons to suit your individual needs.

PLAYING FAVORITES AND
FACING THE UNFAMILIAR

Among the lessons in the Change Your Age Program, pick half a dozen that you found the most enjoyable or interesting and string them together for a program of your own design. You can learn about yourself by seeing which lessons feel most pleasurable to you and which ones feel difficult. By now, you've probably discovered that some of the lessons came easily or naturally to you and others were more confusing or challenging, perhaps evoking resistance in your back or knees. Be sure to differentiate between a feeling of uncertainty, on the one hand, and stiffness and actual pain, on the other. Don't challenge yourself through pain.

Although it is tempting to stick with your favorite lessons, a useful challenge would be to construct a routine made up of your least favorite lessons. After all, it could be these lessons that will keep your brain the fittest and your body most able to do more difficult and unfamiliar movements. It's important to realize that some movements will feel natural to one person and awkward to the next. It could be that a movement that makes you feel uncoordinated simply hasn't yet entered the realm of the familiar for you.

Usually what feels most comfortable, easy, and acceptable to people are the movements that are also most deeply ingrained and habitual. These preferences can be limiting. You can get used to turning your head only a few degrees to the left or right, you can become accustomed to not being able to raise your arms high over your head, and you can find it comfortable to get out of a chair by pushing with your arms and holding your breath, but these adaptations to the familiar can become the basis for narrower and ever more restricted ways of moving as we age. If you want to expand and vary the ways in which you move and have more complete and easier access to your environment, it's important to practice the unfamiliar and the nonhabitual.

Remember that variations of movement through tendons, ligaments, muscles, and joints not only are good for the structures of your body but also greatly benefit the functioning of your mind. Just as a lack of variation causes limitations in our joints, so it causes limitations in our feelings—and imagination. Ultimately, stiffness and lack of physical imagination lead to the appearance and actuality of premature aging.

Here is a way of understanding the difference between the habitual and the nonhabitual. Interlace the fingers of your two hands and notice if the feeling in your hands is familiar and comfortable. Then, with your eyes closed, uncross your hands and recross them with the opposite thumb and index finger on top. Many people find that they have to open their eyes to see which thumb and index finger are on top. When people cross their fingers in the opposite and unfamiliar way, their hands feel awkward. Another example is to cross your arms and observe which one is on top. If you uncross your arms and recross them with the other one on top, it might feel confusing, particularly if you do this with your eyes closed. You can expand the ways in which you move and how your brain maps movement by exploring movements that feel unfamiliar.

Again, practice movements that you don't prefer as well as the ones that make you feel most comfortable. Remember that most of the lessons can be done with your eyes closed. You can also return to the State of the Body Scan at any time during or between the lessons.

HOW MANY REPETITIONS SHOULD I DO?

Whether you construct your own routine or choose one of the routines given in this chapter, give yourself time to do the most important thing—feel what you are doing and shine a brighter light on your awareness of the movement. For example, doing 20 repetitions of the same movement can become stressful to your tendons, ligaments, and joints. On the other hand, doing three movements or fewer will probably provide too little physical information to deepen your sense of how you're performing the movement. One of the things you will be learning is the right balance between too hard and too easy, between too much and not enough.

HOW OFTEN SHOULD I PRACTICE THE CHANGE YOUR AGE LESSONS?

As I recommend to my clients, I suggest limiting your time doing these movements when you start. Don't spend more than 30 minutes a day doing these movements. Try to do them every day, but if you can't, try them fewer times a week—say, three to five times. The important thing is that you do the lessons every week. After a while, you may find yourself wanting to perform them for a half-hour or more each day. To receive their full transformational potential, do these movements slowly and with full attention.

HOW FAST SHOULD I MOVE?

Your speed of motion will tend to decline as you age. However, practicing new movements until you can perform them adeptly and quickly can develop a different sense of yourself in motion. Your brain records variations in speed by involving more cells; it's most important that you start slowly and take your time while you are learning. Faster movement will then become automatic and you will counteract the tendency to move more slowly as you age.

The best way to transform your movements and adjust your movement quotient is to use your imagination. Many of the movements in this program can be performed by getting into the starting position, actually doing one or two movements slowly, and then imagining how you would do the movement. As you imagine doing the movement, your mind goes into motion but your body remains at rest in the starting position. This is one of the most powerful ways to improve at any activity.

Imagining how you would do a movement and then physically returning to the movement can create more improvement than repeating the action many times. Mindless repetition of a movement won't create the necessary transformation that could occur with each of these lessons. Stopping and repeating, like a mental rehearsal, enables you to have more success and helps you tune in to the details that your brain needs to help your muscles and bones perform with greater ease.

MORNING ROUTINE

The morning routine provided here is a good way to start your day. The goal of this sequence is to gently and gradually awaken your mind and body by taking you from the floor to standing in a series of easy-to-do lessons that flow in a way that you could use every day. Soon you will find all of the lessons easier to do.

Some people do their exercises in the morning first thing, even before drinking a cup of coffee, because that helps to set their coordination for the rest of the day. However, this routine—an ideal way to move from the floor to standing—is one you could do any time of the day.

After learning this sequence thoroughly, do it once each morning as a refreshing way to wake up. Remember, it's okay to leave out any movements you find difficult or impossible to do. Once you've learned this routine, each lesson in it will take about three minutes to perform. If you find this combination of lessons too long for your morning schedule, feel free to pick and choose from this routine. Remember, variety is important, so each day you can make different selections.

Lesson 1: Coordinating Your Neck and Eyes with Your Legs and Pelvis
Lesson 2: Releasing the Hips into Pleasure
Lesson 5: Rolling into Length Across Your Stomach
Lesson 8: The Middle of the Body: Expanding, Reaching, and Turning
Lesson 10: Turning from Your Pelvis
Lesson 15: Moving from the Chair to the Floor and Returning
Lesson 20: Crawling with Your Knees Up and Down
Lesson 21: Upright Kneeling
Lesson 22: Through Crouching to Standing
Lesson 25: Freeing Stiff Hips and Knees
Lesson 26: Improving Balance
Lesson 28: Standing on the Highest Point of the Hip

ENERGIZING ROUTINE

This routine is an effective way to pick up the tempo if you are feeling sluggish and need to develop a little more tone. I suggest doing this at any time of the day, though not before you are trying to go to sleep.

After you've gotten comfortable with these lessons, try performing them at a higher speed. Continue to start Lesson 6 and its Advanced Variations, as well as Lesson 17, slowly, but then begin to speed up for Lessons 18 to 30. After you perform the routine once through, you can continue to maintain a higher cardiovascular output by repeating the sequence from Lesson 24 to Lesson 30.

You can build the energizing routine into any other exercise activity you enjoy. After anything from a stroll to a run, you can use the lessons in the Energizing Routine to improve your flexibility, balance, and coordination.

MIDDAY ROUTINE

The lessons in the midday routine are designed to be done sitting in a chair. Most of us do have to sit each day, so this routine will give you a change of pressure, loosen your ligaments, oil your joints, and lengthen your muscles. You can do most of these lessons at work and inspire any other people who may be watching. After all, you are changing your age.

Since many people spend hours upon hours sitting in a chair each day, it's good to be able to move easily in your chair. Think of how a child looks at and relates to a chair, seeing it perhaps as a fort or a jungle gym. Becoming an adult involves sitting still and paying attention, which can lead to rigidity in our muscles and tendons, pain in our head, neck, and shoulders, and especially pain in our lower back. Many people find that it's harder to sit for a prolonged period of time than to stand or walk. In fact, the pressures on the spine are greater in sitting than standing. Because there is continuous movement throughout our spines when we stand or walk, these actions can give us a feeling of relief from pressure. *An alternative way of relieving the pressure of sitting is to lie on the floor and do any of the lessons in the lying-down position (Chapter 3, Lessons 1 to 9).*

FITNESS BOOST

These lessons put enough pressure on your bones and skeleton to seriously improve your bone density. They require pressures and forces that are healthy for your bones, your ligaments, and the muscles close to your joints. The insides of your bones grow in density and strength in response to the stress of your muscles pulling or in response to gravity pulling down.

For example, if you stand high on your hip joint, you are putting pressure and force directly on your femur, or thighbone. Exerting pressure down on the femur will lead to greater growth and density in the hip bone (see Lesson 28). If you stand with your hip jutting out to the side, however, you are exerting pressure to the side and not encouraging as much growth in the bone density of the hip-joint socket and the head, or ball, of the femur. So the higher the point of your hip joint that you stand on, the more solid or dense the hip joint grows inside.

The Fitness Boost exercises suggested here require using your strongest antigravity muscles, which are the large strong muscles of the back, hips, and thighs that prevent us from falling over, or, if you will, being pushed down by gravity. By activating the core muscles of your body—that is, the muscles deep inside and closest to your joints, the ones you can't see so easily—you'll feel more stable and stronger.

Weight-bearing exercises are best for strengthening. Swimming is good for growing muscles, but it doesn't foster as much bone growth because it doesn't exert as much force on the bones as weight lifting, running, or tennis. Resistance exercises, like weight lifting, have repeatedly demonstrated that they promote the growth of bones, along with muscles.

As you get involved in this new movement program and become stronger, you will discover changes in all layers of your body. You aren't just adding muscle on top of your bones—your bones must grow to keep up with your muscles. Then your brain has to recalibrate and recoordinate the way you move with a sturdier, less fragile body.

As with the other routines, learn these lessons thoroughly before combining them in these sequences or adding them to your current strength and fitness program. If you have an exercise program or sport you enjoy, try rotating that program with the lessons in this section, or from anywhere in the book.

Lesson 17: Baby Alligator
Lesson 19: Finding the Two Halves of Your Body
Lesson 24: Crouching for Your Life
Lesson 28: Standing on the Highest Point of the Hip
Lesson 29: Jumping to Discover Your Posture
Advanced Variation on Lesson 29: Jumping to Discover Your Posture
Lesson 30: Hopping for Health

NIGHTTIME ROUTINES

At night, when you want to wind down, the lessons in this routine will help release you from the stresses of the day, give you the opportunity to return from upright posture to the ground, and prepare you for a relaxing evening or, if you are close to bedtime, for sleep.

Remember to perform the movements slowly and to let your breathing direct the pace of your movements. You can do many of these lessons with your eyes closed, which will increase sensory awareness of your body and calm you down even more. Rest on your back between each of these lessons and do a brief State of the Body Scan.

Lesson 3: Using Your Abdomen to Release Your Back
Lesson 7: A Simple Rolling Lesson

SLEEP ENHANCEMENT TIPS

Many people find that the slower, softer movements in the Change Your Age Program help them fall asleep, probably because these movements reduce stress and discomfort in areas of our bodies that are ordinarily excluded from exercise programs. But the greater body awareness that arises from following the program can also yield a more active dream state.

Many people who are restless sleepers, including those with RLS (restless leg syndrome), report these lessons having a calming effect. The key to a good night's sleep is to create a shift in your autonomic or vegetative nervous system.

Your autonomic nervous system, which controls everything from your blood pressure to your digestive system and your heart rate, can create feelings from intense arousal and stress to profound calmness and relaxation. The autonomic nervous system is divided into two parts: the sympathetic system and the parasympathetic system. It's through the sympathetic system that you experience the "fight or flight" reaction: Your muscles contract, the openings of your interior organs shut down, your heart speeds up, your arteries constrict, and you become hyper-alert and ready for action.

This kind of hyper-arousal can happen to any of us very quickly. For example, you might be startled by a vehicle suddenly appearing and barely missing you while you're crossing a street, or maybe you jump when you suddenly hear a loud sound close to you; perhaps you've woken with a start when you remember something. Your body reacts quickly and reflexively in such circumstances and throws your entire system into a stress-ready state.

Although you can quickly become aroused and reactive to danger, you can't go as quickly from hyper-arousal to falling asleep. It takes time to alter this state, which happens through the other branch of the autonomic nervous system—the parasympathetic system.

The parasympathetic system dilates the pupils of your eyes, dilates your intestines and stomach so you can digest food, slows down the speed of your heart, and allows you to lower the pressures inside your body, creating an ideal internal environment for deep relaxation or sleep.

It takes longer for the parasympathetic system to act. The sympathetic nervous system is set up as a chain of ganglia, or bundles of nerves, along your spine and through your body. When these nerves fire, they all fire at once—it's all or nothing. By contrast, the parasympathetic system comprises ganglia that are situated all over the body and divided from each other. Therefore, stimulation of one bundle of nerves does not set off a chain reaction; instead, the parasympathetic system is activated slowly, piece by piece.

The lessons in the following routine, like all the lessons in this book, will help you shift into the parasympathetic state of your autonomic nervous system, leaving you feeling more relaxed overall.

You may want to blend your bedtime preparation activities—brushing your teeth, changing into pajamas, checking the doors or turning off the lights—with any or all of the movements in this routine.

The routine doesn't have to be performed in sequence; feel free to use any of the lessons alone or in combination to reduce the stress of your day and get a better night's sleep. Be sure to include a lesson on your back, stomach, or side that will make it easier for you to sleep in your favorite positions.

Lesson 2, "Releasing the Hips into Pleasure," helps many people to sleep by releasing tightness around the hips and legs.

Lesson 3, "Using Your Abdomen to Release Your Back," frees your back for a better night's sleep and helps prevent morning back pain.

Lesson 4, "Seesaw Breathing," keeps your rib cage and the muscles used for breathing limber for nighttime sleep.

Lesson 5, "Rolling into Length Across Your Stomach," is a good lesson to perform if you find it difficult to sleep on your stomach.

Lesson 7, "A Simple Rolling Lesson," is a good way to start your nighttime routine.

DEVELOPING A MORE EXPRESSIVE FACE: REDUCING TENSION IN YOUR JAW, MOUTH, FACE, AND NECK

In addition to the benefits of these lessons, you might find that relaxing the unconscious tensions in your jaw, upper neck, and face promotes better sleep. I have developed a program to reduce temporomandibular joint (TMJ) stress that can occur in the jaw joint and that contributes significantly to bruxism, or teeth grinding at night while asleep. Overnight teeth grinding reveals that your sympathetic nervous system is still firing. By learning to relax your jaw, you can give your sympathetic system a break and shift more easily to the parasympathetic system—and find yourself getting a better night's sleep.

If you tighten your jaw too much, it's extremely likely that you will have a very tight neck and back muscles as well. For example, if you clench your teeth, you might feel some strain in your neck. Try lifting this book and moving it around while your teeth are tightly fastened together. Now stop, relax your jaw, and think about yawning, which relaxes the throat muscles. Lift the book again and notice whether the book feels lighter and lifting it is easier. If you tighten your jaw while standing, you are likely to feel muscles in your lower back and belly contracting and your neck shortening.

The following lesson will show you how to improve the function of your mouth and jaw so that movement is more comfortable and any muscular stress or tension in your jaw, mouth, face, or neck is reduced. The head, neck, and jaw are common sites for pain. You may have a problem that requires the attention of a dentist or oral surgeon, but supplementing medical intervention with this exercise can bring you added relief.

This lesson calls for gentle movements of the eyes, face, and tongue, integrated with the jaw. Stress in any of these areas can affect the jaw. This lesson will allow you to more easily use your jaw by breaking up rigid and painful patterns of work in all the muscles of the mouth, jaw, face, and neck. Many people also find that this lesson improves the expressivity of their face, makes it easier to breathe more comfortably, and even improves their voice.

If you have difficulties with any of the movements of this lesson, learn to do them both sitting and lying. Also, the effectiveness of the lesson depends on how slowly and attentively you do the movements—not on the number of repetitions. The more slowly you do the movements, the easier they will become. Having a sense of ease and comfort is the most important thing. If you feel pain, make the movements smaller and produce the movements with less effort.

The intention of this lesson is to reveal how the muscles involved in facial expression act in harmony with the movements of the jaw. If the muscles of your lips, cheeks, and the rest of your face do not move, it is also more difficult for your jaw to move freely.

This lesson would be most beneficial if done both lying on your back on the floor (or on your bed) and sitting upright on the floor or in a chair. Always begin by practicing the lesson sitting in a chair. The more positions you find in which you can practice this movement, the more your unconscious mind will release the tightness in the muscles of your jaw.

1. Put the index and middle fingers of one hand just below your ear and find the hinge of your jaw. With your eyes closed, open and close your jaw slightly to help find the hinge. Slide your jaw from side to side as well. Can you feel it with your fingers?

2. Glide your jaw forward and backward. Do you feel more strain in your throat or neck while doing this movement? Can your lips facilitate the gliding movement?

3. Stop moving your jaw and instead move your lips forward and back. How does this movement affect your jaw? Reach your lips forward in a round "O" shape, as if you were reaching your lips to kiss someone. Can you feel your jaw glide forward automatically?

4. Now slowly pull your lips so far back that you find yourself with a big grin on your face. If you slowly smile, you will feel your jaw retract. The bigger your smile, the greater the motion of your jaw. Can you feel your jaw gliding backward?

5. Alternate between reaching your lips forward in a big kiss and backward in a big wide smile, feeling your jaw gliding forward and back with the movements of your lips. Allow your neck to participate in this back-and-forth motion.

Change Your Age Tip: In a seated position, allow your head to glide forward with your jaw as you reach your lips forward, and then let the back of your head move backward as you move your lips and jaw back into a grin. For many people who have difficulties, this movement of the face and head can unlock the jaw.

The forward and backward action of the jaw is primarily related to the kissing and smiling functions of the face. These movements are not necessary to chew food, but all primates must be able to make these social gestures of the face and jaw to survive in their community. You could say that the forward and backward motions of the jaw and face are social movements. The forward and backward action of the head in harmony with these motions of the jaw and face is also seen in the walking of most birds and mammals, most visibly the chicken and the horse.

6. Learn to do this movement of the lips, jaw, and head fairly lightly and quickly after you have mastered it by going very slowly. Also, try turning your head to either side and performing the same movement while aimed in a different direction.

    Rest and observe the feeling of your face, mouth, jaw, and neck. Notice where your head sits on top of your spine. When you stand up and walk, notice whether your head responds to the movement of your legs. If not, can you create such a response?

● ● ●

IN THIS chapter, we have looked at some of the ways in which you can customize the Change Your Age Program to suit a variety of your needs. Remember, you don't have to do all 30 lessons to benefit from the program. Breaking up the lessons into shorter sequences for different purposes can help you more easily integrate the program into your everyday life.

The next chapter will show you how to examine some limitations on your movement that could be related to specific signs of aging and their associated aches and pains—and how the Change Your Age Program can help alleviate any such problems.

CHAPTER FIVE

USING THE PROGRAM IN YOUR EVERYDAY LIFE

How to Transform Your Habits to Avoid Pain and Injury

IT IS useful to alter our perceptions of pain. If we look at pain as a limitation on our mobility, we can address pain issues by changing the way we move.

The Change Your Age Program is not a pain management program; it is a program to help you move more easily and more youthfully. But by changing how you move, you will find that you can manage your pain and lessen the chance of injury.

Pain, stiffness, fatigue—these are issues that affect us all as we age. But if we reframe how we look at pain, stiffness, and fatigue, we can come to understand them as the result of bad postural, movement, timing, and balance habits. This chapter revisits the Change Your Age Mobility Survey from Chapter 2 and offers suggestions that will help you transform your habits and feel better fast, some lessons from Chapter 3 that can help you relearn your habits, and some inspiring success stories. Don't feel that you need to follow all of these suggestions. Consider them a resource you can turn to when necessary.

POSTURAL HABITS

Almost every day I hear the question, "What is good posture?" To me, this question reveals that posture is difficult to think about and difficult to feel.

You may think about posture in the standard way: as the bones of your body being stacked up like bricks and your balance and mechanical alignment being ideally expressed with your head in a precise position above your chest, which is in a precise position above your pelvis, and so on, down to your feet on the floor.

You can stand in this kind of alignment, like a breathless etiquette teacher with a book balanced on her head, but the difficulty with this concept of posture is that it does not allow you to move very easily and your breathing becomes strained.

Your body cannot be compared to a stack of bricks or a building because you have a brain. And your brain determines your posture. What you sense, what you are feeling at any particular moment, your intentions—all of these things determine your posture. No one just stands up for no reason—we all stand up *for* something. Our posture contains our entire emotional history: We learned to stand up as infants to do something, and we learned finally to form a personality so we could stand up for ourselves. Our self-image, our ego, and our intentions to perform actions determine our posture, not some abstract and artificial ideas based on mechanical alignment.

Good posture while you are standing and talking intimately to a good friend or your lover is quite different—and rightly so—from the posture you have when talking to someone you've never met before or someone you feel threatened by. What would be the ideal posture for being prepared to receive a tennis serve? What would be the ideal posture for a quarterback who is about to receive the ball from the center and intends to make a long pass? Good posture is being able to adapt our posture to many situations and to use it to express who we are socially.

So perhaps a better question than "What is good posture?"—as if posture were a static sort of thing—would be: "What is the range of postural possibilities?" How adaptable is your posture to different situations? If your posture creates pain, then you need to move differently inside of yourself and not stand like a stack of bricks.

A CHANGE YOUR AGE SUCCESS STORY

Susan had appeared in my studio unable to straighten one of her knees. She was told that she would need a knee replacement, which she very much wanted to avoid. It was only when she insisted on avoiding surgery that her physician suggested that she visit me.

At our first meeting, Susan explained why it was logical that her knee problem was a problem only with her knee and why the only solution for her would be surgery. She demonstrated this by limping around the room. I pointed out that she was overusing her other leg, she had to distort the movements of her pelvis and back, and in fact she was becoming stiff all over—all because she was afraid of damaging her knee further and then having to face the surgery she did not want to undergo.

I worked with her, through movement and touch, for several sessions until she learned to re-sense how she could straighten her knee, how to awaken new muscles, and how to walk in a new way that would de-stress her knee and, in fact, de-stress much of her body. I asked Susan for a commitment to a program in which she would learn how to reorganize her posture. The way she compressed her head and neck and drew her shoulders forward and up was visibly affecting the pressure going down through her hips and into her knees. As I worked with her, her chest became more elevated and her shoulders lowered and became broader. There was now room for her neck to be longer. As she walked, I asked her how she felt now. She said, "It's strange—it feels as if I had a sack on my head pushing me down, and now that it's gone I feel less strain in my knee."

I also worked with the tightness around her jaw. Susan had been grinding her teeth at night for many years. It's very common for anyone who tightens the jaw too much to also have a very tight neck and back muscles. As Susan was able to relax her throat and jaw, her breathing became easier and her lower back and hips became freer.

Though people often don't make the connection, the habit of tightening parts of the upper body supports the habit of not being able to move the lower body well, and vice versa. For example, your entire body reacts if you stub your toe. In fact, many people develop an acute back spasm or find that their neck becomes extremely tight. Reflexive reactions to pain spread throughout our whole body. Usually they disappear shortly after the painful event, but we are very capable of wearing our habits—as though putting on a raincoat and forgetting it is a sunny day—and so we hold on to our tight neck and back or maintain a look like we are waiting to exhale. We maintain these habits until they become part of our character.

Susan found it much easier to move her knees, improve her balance, and de-stress both of her legs before I ever touched them by changing her tense upper body and tightly slumped posture.

Susan still hasn't had her surgery and now takes dance classes, goes for long walks with her dog, and practices her new ways to move. Whenever she needs a reminder, she makes another appointment to get some fresh Change Your Age tips.

● ● ●

1. DO YOU HAVE DIFFICULTY TURNING YOUR HEAD FROM SIDE TO SIDE?

Sometimes postural difficulties make it difficult to turn the head. The ability to scan the environment easily requires upright posture and freedom of motion in the neck.

How to Transform Your Habits
Lie on the floor with your legs extended long and slowly roll your head from side to side. Make sure your jaw is relaxed. Take a deep breath, relax your shoulders and your jaw, and look at something in front of yourself as you turn your head from one side to the other. Feel that the motion of your head

is separate from the motion of your eyes. If you can, when you take your head a little to the right, take your eyes a little to the left, so that your head and your eyes go in opposite directions.

Take another deep breath, pause, and notice whether your head turns more freely.

See the following lessons:

Lesson 1: Coordinating Your Neck and Eyes with Your Legs and Pelvis
Lesson 6: Regaining Full Use of Your Neck
Lesson 7: A Simple Rolling Lesson
Lesson 8: The Middle of the Body: Expanding, Reaching, and Turning
Lesson 10: Turning from Your Pelvis
Lesson 17: Baby Alligator

2. DO YOU HAVE DIFFICULTY CLIMBING UP AND DOWN STAIRS?

As we age, both our hips and knees tend to stay slightly bent, limiting the length of our stride. This can, of course, interfere with our ability to climb up and down stairs. We must be able to extend our hip backward and straighten our knees if we are to have the full use of the upright gait that has evolved in humans.

How to Transform Your Habits

Exaggerate your gait by acting like a chimpanzee. Bend your knees more than you are used to and then straighten them. Look out at the horizon. Bend and straighten your knees slowly several times, and then do it quickly, as if you were about to jump. If your heels leave the floor when you come up, that's good. Do the same movement, pushing harder through one leg and then the other, until you push more quickly and bend more quickly through either leg.

Practicing bending and extending your knees as if you were going to jump will help you climb your stairs and increase the length of your stride.

See the following lessons:

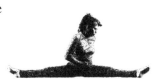

3. DO YOU HAVE LABORED OR SHALLOW BREATHING?

Labored or shallow breathing often results when a slumped posture con-stricts the diaphragm. This is a strong habit reinforced by either a lack of or too rigid an extension through the whole body. People curve their spine for-ward and are unable to straighten their hips and knees completely or they are rigidly extended so they cannot move their ribs freely.

How to Transform Your Habits

Inhale a small amount of air. Hold your breath. Without letting any air in or out, raise your chest as if you were pulling the air up higher in your lungs. Next push that air down into your lower belly and even into your lower back. Your chest will go down. Every so often, in any position—sitting, standing, or, best of all, lying down—inhale a small amount of air, hold your breath, and pass the imaginary ball of air down into your pelvis and up to the top of your chest.

Notice whether you breathe more easily after doing this.

See the following lessons:

4. DO YOU HAVE A PROTRUDING ABDOMEN AND AN OVERLY ARCHED BACK?

A protruding abdomen is not the result of weak stomach muscles but is more often a postural issue related to how we organize and coordinate the movements of our back, hips, arms, and legs. A fuller, upright posture allows the weight of the belly to be carried by the bony basin of the pelvis, an anatomical design feature unique to humans.

How to Transform Your Habits

Sit in the middle of a chair with your feet directly under your knees. Push down through your legs only enough to bounce your pelvis forward, toward the front of the chair, and then backward a little farther, toward the back of the chair.

With your hands on your belly, tilt backward in the chair a little bit until you feel the muscles in your stomach contract. Tilt forward and backward a few times and feel how your stomach muscles engage in support of the belly.

Put your hands on your waist or your stomach to feel how those muscles work as you bounce your pelvis forward and backward.

See the following lessons:

Lesson 3: Using Your Abdomen to Release Your Back

Advanced Variation on Lesson 3: Using Your Abdomen to Release Your Back

Lesson 4: Seesaw Breathing

Lesson 16: Jump-Sitting in a Chair

Advanced Variation on Lesson 16: Jump-Sitting on the Floor

Lesson 28: Standing on the Highest Point of the Hip

Lesson 29: Jumping to Discover Your Posture

5. DO YOU HAVE A SLUMPED POSTURE?

A slumped posture indicates a curvature of the spine. The forward head position, tight neck, and depressed chest that result make it difficult to hold the face up.

How to Transform Your Habits

While standing, can you reach one arm up toward the ceiling or the sky? Look at your hand and keep reaching until you feel your outstretched arm lifting your ribs. Make sure your jaw stays open. Put your arm down and do the same with the other arm. Let the reach occur as if someone were pulling you up higher through that arm. Your heels might come off the floor. Then simply stand and notice how much taller you feel. As you walk, you can always be prepared to reach up and point to the sky.

See the following lessons:

Lesson 4: Seesaw Breathing
Lesson 5: Rolling into Length Across Your Stomach
Lesson 6: Regaining Full Use of Your Neck
Lesson 7: A Simple Rolling Lesson
Lesson 8: The Middle of the Body: Expanding, Reaching, and Turning
Lesson 13: Chair Play
Lesson 14: The Sitting and Turning Dance
Lesson 16: Jump-Sitting in a Chair
Lesson 27: The Ultimate Walking Lesson
Lesson 29: Jumping to Discover Your Posture
Lesson 30: Hopping for Health

MOVEMENT HABITS

Most of the 30 basic exercises could be formulated out of the startle reflex: the movements that occur when we react to a sudden, unexpected stimulus. In four-fifths of a second, we quickly use all of our muscles, from our back out to our fingertips, to extend ourselves fully, and our eyes take on a look of surprise and hypervigilance. Then we pull in and down into a semicrouch: Our chin tucks down to protect our throat, and our chest moves down to protect our diaphragm. We tighten and harden our stomach and the inside of our legs as we grab the ground with our feet (even in high-heeled shoes). We remain hypervigilant and embrace our body to ward off possible impending blows.

Many people remain in one half or the other of the startle reflex all the time. Stress induces the startle pattern, which is popularly called the fight-or-flight response but could more accurately be described as "fight, flight, or what?" A lack of confidence can be built into the posture. Sometimes when people are least expecting it, a situation triggers the thoughts and feelings that lead, in whole or in part, to the expression of this startle response.

Along with the movement habits associated with the startle response are the neural and chemical responses. Our body is immediately awash with adrenaline, cortical steroids, and almost 50 other chemical agents that our organs manufacture to keep us excited and ready for action. The startle reflex causes our pupils to constrict, almost stops the blood flow to our digestive organs, increases our heart rate, and intensifies the internal pressures from all of our organs and muscles. This is not only a state designed for very specific circumstances but a state that can be great fun if you are moving fast, enjoying the activity you're engaged in, and in need of quick bursts of energy, which, once released and acted upon, can leave you feeling quite calm afterward. But this stress state was not designed to be maintained for a prolonged period of time. It's okay to strongly contract your back or stomach, but it's not good to hold on to your back and stomach day after day, for weeks, months, or years. Eventually these deep habits will begin to distort your body.

In spite of the strength of these ancient reflexes and in spite of the stresses of life—many of which are healthy, enjoyable, motivating, and otherwise worthwhile—we can and must learn to develop ourselves and mature beyond the limitations set by the reflexes we were born with. As we get older, we retain a strong ability to keep learning new things. Indeed, we now know that the human brain can reengineer many of its features.

As I've emphasized throughout, the best way to break through restrictive boundaries is to explore and discover new ways to move. Babies have to do it every day, all day. All humans learn to walk, to sing, to dance, by first learning new ways to move. Think of any skill you ever acquired in your entire life-time, and you can appreciate the fact that you acquired that skill by altering and redesigning your habits.

A CHANGE YOUR AGE SUCCESS STORY

Elizabeth was sitting at the dinner table one Sunday night and reaching with a spoon to feed her baby. It fell on the floor between them, and as she bent over to pick it up from the floor, in a diagonally reaching movement, she felt as if something in her back snapped. She was barely able to sit back up again and was in acute pain. Her husband had to help her get out of the chair and carry her to the bed, where she lay for hours.

Elizabeth was not only in pain but also confused. To her friends, she had been a role model for how to go through pregnancy pain-free and in good shape. She had continued to take yoga classes and do exercises until she went into labor, and she returned to these activities soon after giving birth. Now her child was a year old, and it seemed inconceivable that she could injure her back by bending over to pick up plastic dinnerware. After having an X-ray and an MRI, she was told that she had a herniated lower lumbar disk, but the doctors did not suggest any form of back operation. Instead, they gave her an epidural to stop the pain, told her to limit her movements and wait and see what happened.

When Elizabeth came to see me, she warned me that she couldn't really be moved and that she had been learning to just bend her knees, not her back. She had some idea that she should stay that way.

I placed a ball on the floor just next to and in front of where she was sitting. I wanted to know where the spoon was in relation to her body when she bent over to pick it up. Following that direction, I had her do a series of slow, easy movements, massaging up and down her legs, remaining inside the range that was comfortable. She then explored a variety of ways of bending that were comfortable. Sometimes her brain could not allow her to move farther until she had changed her breathing habits, thus increasing her range of comfort.

I showed Elizabeth new and unfamiliar ways of turning her trunk while she bent forward and helped her find a better place to put her feet so that her legs could do most of the work of bending over and returning. Within half an hour, she discovered that she could make a diagonal reach to the floor, pick up the ball, and hand it to me.

Elizabeth was amazed that this movement did not hurt. I asked her to sit with her feet out of place, in an awkward position, and to hold her breath a little bit. I put the ball back on the floor and asked her to pick it up again while wearing her old set of habits. Immediately, her back began to hurt again. So she stopped, repositioned her feet, and took a deep breath. She imagined picking up the ball comfortably and slowly, until she could clearly feel in her mind how she would contract her legs, use her pressure against the floor, and keep breathing. Once again, she was able to pick up the ball without pain. Elizabeth realized that she now had control over her back pain. By understanding how she could *intentionally* make her pain worse, she realized how she could also make it better.

● ● ●

6.   DO YOUR MOVEMENTS FEEL HEAVY, AS IF SOMEONE TURNED UP THE GRAVITY?

When we are feeling stressed, anxious, or overworked, the muscles on both sides of our joints contract. For example, if your back muscles contract from the back and your chest and belly muscles contract from the front, your spine will become compressed. However, you can learn your way out of these ancient and habitual stress reactions.

How to Transform Your Habits

For a few seconds, exaggerate the feeling of being pushed down from the top and being tight in the torso, as if a bag of sand were on your head. Now take the imaginary sandbag off your head and feel the length and lightness in your posture when you're not scrunched up. Make a daily practice of performing this movement of feeling squashed down and tight in your torso and neck and then releasing it.

See the following lessons:

Lesson 1: Coordinating Your Neck and Eyes with Your Legs and Pelvis
Lesson 2: Releasing the Hips into Pleasure
Lesson 4: Seesaw Breathing
Lesson 7: A Simple Rolling Lesson
Lesson 8: The Middle of the Body: Expanding, Reaching, and Turning
Lesson 9: Crossed-Arm, Crossed-Ankle Foot Lifting—Advanced
    Lying Lesson
Lesson 13: Chair Play
Lesson 14: The Sitting and Turning Dance
Lesson 16: Jump-Sitting in a Chair
Lesson 25: Freeing Stiff Hips and Knees
Lesson 27: The Ultimate Walking Lesson
Lesson 29: Jumping to Discover Your Posture
Lesson 30: Hopping for Health

7. DO YOU COMPLAIN OF HAVING A STIFF LOWER BACK AND TIGHT HIPS?

Many people tighten their lower back and restrict the freedom of motion in their pelvis because it feels awkward and exaggerated to let their pelvis and back move as much as they could. This is a deeply ingrained habit. If people in Ohio could learn to sway their hips like people in Brazil, their lower backs would be much less stiff!

How to Transform Your Habits

When your back feels stiff, lie on the floor, bend your knees, and stand your feet wide apart. Relax your breathing and relax your jaw. Put your arms wherever they're comfortable.

Push gently through your feet until your pelvis begins to roll toward your head and you feel your lower back getting closer to the floor. Release this movement and roll your pelvis the other way, toward your feet. Go back and forth, rolling your pelvis, from head to foot. Keep your neck and jaw feeling free so that your head also moves.

You can do this movement slowly, but sometimes do it lightly and easily, with a rhythm. Let yourself breathe more and more.

See the following easy lessons:

Lesson 1: Coordinating Your Neck and Eyes with Your Legs and Pelvis
Lesson 2: Releasing the Hips into Pleasure
Lesson 3: Using Your Abdomen to Release Your Back
Lesson 4: Seesaw Breathing
Lesson 5: Rolling into Length Across Your Stomach
Lesson 7: A Simple Rolling Lesson

Consider also including these more difficult but effective lessons:

Lesson 10: Turning from Your Pelvis
Lesson 11: Developing Longer Hamstrings the Easy Way
Lesson 12: Oiling Your Hips the Easy Way
Lesson 17: Baby Alligator
Lesson 20: Crawling with Your Knees Up and Down
Lesson 22: Through Crouching to Standing
Lesson 23: How to Approach Squatting
Lesson 24: Crouching for Your Life
Lesson 25: Freeing Stiff Hips and Knees
Lesson 26: Improving Balance

8. DO YOU GET ANXIOUS ABOUT YOUR BALANCE WHEN YOU REACH UP OR LOOK UP?

Many people don't notice that they have balance difficulties until they are placed in a situation where balance can be an issue. When you're looking up, the vestibular system in your inner ear can give you an unfamiliar sensation that doesn't happen when you reach your arm over your head while still looking forward. That unfamiliar sensation can create anxiety.

How to Transform Your Habits

Stand with your right foot crossed over your left foot. Look up as if reaching for something. Reach with one arm and then the other. Let your pelvis move in the opposite direction that you reach. Repeat this movement with your left foot on the outside of your right foot. Reach all around yourself, in every possible direction, and feel how your pelvis and feet support you. Remember to breathe and feel your breathing while you're doing this. Smile!

See the following lessons:

Lesson 6: Regaining Full Use of Your Neck
Lesson 7: A Simple Rolling Lesson
Variation on Lesson 7: Simple Rolling from Side-Lying to Sitting
Lesson 8: The Middle of the Body: Expanding, Reaching, and Turning

See also these more advanced lessons:

Lesson 9: Crossed-Arm, Crossed-Ankle Foot Lifting—Advanced
    Lying Lesson
Lesson 22: Through Crouching to Standing
Lesson 26: Improving Balance

9. DO YOU FIND YOURSELF PUSHING OFF WITH YOUR HANDS TO GET OUT OF A CHAIR?

Pushing off with your hands to get out of a chair instead of using your leg muscles is an example of a lack of ease in moving from one position to another, such as going from sitting to standing and vice versa.

How to Transform Your Habits

Moving from sitting to standing is only part of a full range of movement that allows you to go from squatting to standing and jumping. Sit in the middle of your chair and jump your pelvis forward and back on your chair without using your hands. Then, before you stand up, think that you're going to jump. Don't actually jump—just feel the act of standing from a chair on the way to jumping. It should be a feeling of lightening the load.

See the following lessons:

Lesson 13: Chair Play
Lesson 14: The Sitting and Turning Dance
Lesson 15: Moving from the Chair to the Floor and Returning
Lesson 16: Jump-Sitting in a Chair
Lesson 23: How to Approach Squatting
Lesson 25: Freeing Stiff Hips and Knees
Lesson 26: Improving Balance

10. DO YOU TEND TO STUMBLE OR SHUFFLE WHEN YOU WALK?

A shuffling, stumbling walk suggests a difficulty in lifting your legs and a greater likelihood that your walk will waver from side to side.

How to Transform Your Habits

Go for a practice walk, either in your house or outdoors. Practice aiming your knees in the direction you're going. For instance, aim your knees toward a door on the other side of the room. If you see a tree down the street, aim your knees at the tree. As you begin your walking motion by first bending your knee, you'll find that your hips move more and your feet lift more. It should feel a little bit like marching.

See the following lessons:

Lesson 2: Releasing the Hips into Pleasure
Lesson 6: Regaining Full Use of Your Neck
Lesson 21: Upright Kneeling
Lesson 25: Freeing Stiff Hips and Knees
Lesson 26: Improving Balance

TIMING HABITS

Most movements work well for us because of timing. Like a good joke, a good kick of the ball into the net at the right time is what counts. You could have the biggest muscles or swing a bat in the most graceful and coordinated manner, but if you don't have the timing to connect with the ball, you strike out.

Some people trip over their own feet, not because their hip flexors aren't strong enough or because their balance isn't good enough, but because of timing errors. They may have mistimed their step and have a kind of movement stutter. This feels like a tiny lapse of attention when your brain should be connecting with an action you are performing and instead it ends up disconnected. Movement stutters can happen even to young people in the best of condition. ("Gee, coach, I just didn't see where the ball was going, and I couldn't get there in time," or the famous times when a top-notch football player has grabbed a fumbled ball, gotten up, and run the wrong way.)

There's excellent video documentation of people in their own homes performing movement stutters as if they were intentional. In slow motion, the video reveals micro-movements. You see, for example, that the hand of a person reaching for a glass is wavering left and right. At any moment, in the video frame, you are uncertain as to where her hand is going to end up. A few frames later, you see her hand incompletely supporting the glass, which tips over in her attempt to lift it up while not yet fully grasping it. In another example, a person walks through a doorway and almost half of his body strikes the frame of the door.

Humans aren't alone in having to deal with movement stutters; these timing difficulties pervade the universe of movement. The great cats, in spite of all their vastly skilled acts of coordination and balance, have been filmed falling head over tail and interrupting graceful sprints. They come up looking ruffled and surprised as they watch their prey walk away.

Movement stutters often make us confused, frustrated, and ashamed because we can't imagine we could be so unfocused or so clumsy. We can learn, however, to control and recoordinate our timing.

Another factor affecting our timing habits is the pace of our movements. As we get older we naturally tend to slow down and to avoid the feeling of acceleration or rapid deceleration. Yet, as many people realize, it may be easier on the knees, hips, and brain to go down stairs more rapidly than more slowly. The slower you go, the more time your muscles have to grasp at your joints. If there are any imbalances in your body, they are more likely to be revealed if you go too slowly.

One of the greatest strains on the lower back and hip joints is to go for a very slow walk. A moderately paced walk stimulates your body's chemistry—including the release of more fluid to lubricate your joints—and provides less of an opportunity for your muscles to overwork trying to balance you. Using some momentum in your stride and a little more speed can be easier on all of your joints, unless you are suffering from a recent injury.

When a comedian is very funny to one part of an audience but not to another, the issue often is about timing. There is no right joke at the wrong time in a social situation. In the same way, there is no correct way to move without considering that all our movements in space are orchestrated in time. I think it is important for everyone to realize that mistiming is also a habit that you have some control over—maybe not with your jokes but definitely with your movements.

A CHANGE YOUR AGE SUCCESS STORY

My client David was a man of moderate size, but he barely fit through the door to my studio. He seemed to be swaying left and right, and his steps seemed to vary in size as he walked forward. But he wasn't doing either of these things: He had movement stutters, which gave the almost imperceptible feeling that he was moving in multiple directions.

David was hesitant about seeing me and uncertain as to what his difficulty was. Specifically, he wanted to learn how to avoid continuously reinjuring his left hand and right knee. He had suffered several injuries to his right knee and had cuts and bruises on his left hand. He was a chef who loved his job but found it difficult and didn't understand why he cut himself so much more than anyone else on his staff. He was trying to understand how his hand injuries were related to banging his right knee against shelves and, as he put it, almost any protruding object that was low enough. David found that this problem was getting worse as he approached 50, and he was afraid it would affect his career at some point in the future.

I had him interlace his fingers and perform gentle and easy, movements that were challenging to his concept of left and right. This required him to focus and develop a richer felt sense of his body so that he could relearn his timing habits and reduce his movement stutters. I directed him to stand with his legs crossed at the ankles and to move his hips from side to side while rocking across his feet. After he learned to do this smoothly with his legs crossed either way, he learned to do it smoothly with his eyes closed, his legs crossed, and his interlaced fingers behind his head as well.

Movements like this physically challenge the sensory system of the brain and place acceptable demands on our ability to sense left and right from the center of our body, down to our feet and up and out to our hands. As David also practiced many of the movements detailed in Chapter 3 of this book, he gradually regained his sense of lateral movement and removed much of his movement stuttering.

This led to a surge of security and well-being in his life. The hesitancy that David expressed in movement stutters had been accompanied by a growing lack of confidence. It was a relief to him to realize that he suffered simply from lack of a particular coordination that he could easily relearn. He stopped cutting his hand and stopped banging his knee. And I enjoyed some gourmet restaurant meals from a confident chef!

● ● ●

11. DO YOU HAVE DIFFICULTY SPEEDING UP YOUR MOVEMENTS?

A problem with speed of movement is often a perceptual problem. As we accelerate, we feel the world rushing past us too quickly. Also, we can't accelerate without eventually decelerating. Both are faster actions that can stress our joints and ligaments if we don't know how to move with greater body awareness.

How to Transform Your Habits

It's important to maintain your body's ability to accelerate. Turn your head from side to side a small amount, but rapidly. Do this just a few times so you don't get dizzy. Look up and down about the same amount and at about the same speed. Get your inner ears familiar with the speed change. Then, when you go for a walk, go to an area that is not crowded with people or cars. Pick a short distance that feels comfortable for you to use to go fast. Swing your arms and let yourself walk as fast as you can, with big steps and a big arm swing. Start with 100 yards. Increase the amount each day. Every so often, turn your head to one side and then the other, while your arms are pumping and you're walking fast.

Practice Lesson 26, "Improving Balance," and Lesson 27, "The Ultimate Walking Lesson," every day. The following lessons will also improve your speed of motion:

Lesson 1: Coordinating Your Neck and Eyes with Your Legs and Pelvis
Lesson 5: Rolling into Length Across Your Stomach
Lesson 12: Oiling Your Hips the Easy Way
Lesson 14: The Sitting and Turning Dance
Lesson 15: Moving from the Chair to the Floor and Returning
Lesson 16: Jump-Sitting in a Chair
Advanced Variation on Lesson 16: Jump-Sitting on the Floor
Lesson 21: Upright Kneeling
Lesson 24: Crouching for Your Life
Lesson 25: Freeing Stiff Hips and Knees

12.   DO YOU FIND THAT YOUR EYES MOVE MORE SLOWLY THAN THEY USED TO?

Moving the eyes quickly can make anyone, of any age, dizzy or nauseous. This tendency, however, reduces your ability to scan the environment, such as when you are looking at traffic before crossing the street.

How to Transform Your Habits

Sit or stand in a relaxed manner. Keep your neck and your jaw feeling soft. Look straight in front of yourself. Slowly move your eyes to a comfortable place to the right, then back again, without moving your head. Do this again, slowly. Then again, but faster. And then a few more times faster still.

Keep your breathing steady. Now walk a little bit. You might feel a different sense of eye speed on the right side.

Repeat this eye movement on the left side, going slower and then faster, until you can go fast.

Finally, with your jaw relaxed and your breathing steady, slowly and calmly move your eyes from right to left, as if scanning the environment. Then do it very fast, without moving your head. Rest.

Now if you turn your head as well as your eyes, you'll find that you can go very quickly.

See the following lessons:

Lesson 8: The Middle of the Body: Expanding, Reaching, and Turning
Lesson 14: The Sitting and Turning Dance
Lesson 17: Baby Alligator
Lesson 24: Crouching for Your Life
Lesson 27: The Ultimate Walking Lesson
Lesson 29: Jumping to Discover Your Posture

13. DO YOU HAVE SLOWER MOVEMENTS AND A SLOWER RESPONSE TIME?

Although slower movements feel safer and can make you feel better about your balance and control as you get older, in fact, learning to move more quickly will make you feel much younger.

How to Transform Your Habits

Practicing the movements suggested in response to the last two questions is a good place to start.

You can also try juggling two tennis balls or bouncing a basketball while you're walking around.

See the following lessons:

Lesson 1: Coordinating Your Neck and Eyes with Your Legs and Pelvis
Lesson 5: Rolling into Length Across Your Stomach
Lesson 6: Regaining Full Use of Your Neck
Advanced Variation A on Lesson 6: Regaining Full Use of Your Neck
More Advanced Variation B on Lesson 6: Regaining Full Use of
    Your Neck
Lesson 14: The Sitting and Turning Dance
Lesson 17: Baby Alligator
Lesson 24: Crouching for Your Life
Lesson 25: Freeing Stiff Hips and Knees
Lesson 27: The Ultimate Walking Lesson

Lesson 29: Jumping to Discover Your Posture
Lesson 30: Hopping for Health

BALANCE HABITS

Inside your inner ear, deep in your skull, are the remnants of seashells, filled with liquid and small, hairlike cilia. This beautiful construction is called the vestibular system. Your vestibular system allows you to know when you are upright or when your head is tilted to one side. The vestibular system is so sensitive to the movement of its own fluids that the slightest change is detectable and requires a reaction. For example, if you turn your head from side to side rapidly, or spin like many children enjoy doing until they get dizzy and fall over, you're stimulating your vestibular system.

As we get older we move more slowly and with fewer radical changes of position, so our vestibular system is less stimulated. This is a visible sign of aging. If you bend over to pick something up, you might do so much more slowly than you did earlier in your life because you have overstimulated your vestibular system. All your muscles have to contract more slowly and your movements have to have less acceleration so that you don't disturb the equilibrium provided by your vestibular system.

Some people as they get older abandon playing their favorite sports or twirling on the dance floor because their vestibular system, and therefore their equilibrium, has been disturbed. A large element of your balance depends on your equilibrium. If you close your eyes while standing on one leg, you'll suddenly feel your vestibular system interacting with all of your muscles in a way that might throw you off balance. That's why most people prefer keeping their eyes open when doing any activity that requires balance. It's extremely valuable to have the input from our vestibular system match up with the input from our other senses, like sight. Perhaps you've experienced the mismatch of sensory input when you are sitting in a stationary car and look out the window at a bus rolling by. You are not in motion, but seeing the bus move can make you feel like you are lurching backward. Ideally, we want our senses to match up—we are more comfortable when our ocular system, our vestibular system, and our neuromuscular system are all aligned.

The best way to get your eyes, inner ear, muscles, and brain working and sensing together is to move in a style similar to the way you moved as an infant and young child. These developmental movements encourage your head to be in many different positions as you roll it to scan with your ears and eyes and move from lying on your stomach, lying on your back, and side-lying to kneeling, crouching, and standing up and balancing. These movements provide a slow, steady, consistent return of what's often lost in our vestibular system as we age.

Working out at the gym, going for a run or a brisk walk, or practicing sports you are familiar with won't help return your vestibular system to the advanced state you developed in your late teenage years; practicing things you already know just locks in established balance habits. To improve the foundation of your movement organization—your balance—you need to refine your habits by exploring new ways to move. You should be cautious if you feel dizzy or nauseous at times, but in the end you will move like a much younger person when you redevelop your vestibular system, which is just as major a body sense as your eyes or the part of the ears used for hearing.

A CHANGE YOUR AGE SUCCESS STORY

Jennifer had experienced several major difficulties in her life that had created so much pain and posed such a threat to her ability to perform at a high level that she was afraid of a rapid decline as she got older. As the head of marketing for a major software design firm, she was used to being in charge, on top, and in complete control of all her faculties. She felt that sleep apnea—a stoppage of breathing and shortage of oxygen to the brain while sleeping—was contributing to a growing list of pain and joint disorders. She had already undergone two surgical procedures on her jaw, had tried every kind of equipment to counteract the apnea, and was now facing the reality that she could hardly walk down the street because she felt tipsy and precarious. Jennifer had difficulty turning her head because doing so gave her feelings of nausea and disequilibrium. When she took her dog for a walk and he pulled on the leash, serious disturbances arose in her back and shoulders. She couldn't imagine standing on one leg anymore and found it a relief just to lie down, but her demanding life had her driving almost an hour each way to work.

Through a combination of gentle, precisely designed movements and touch, Jennifer was able to improve her ability to feel her body and how she was moving. After only a few weeks, her equilibrium began to return. As Jennifer learned how to turn her head, she found that she could do something she had long thought impossible: lying on her stomach with her head turned to one side. Gradually, her balance improved as the sensations of her body, her proprioceptive sense, developed, until finally her inner sensations, which were no longer painful, began to provide the same information to her as her teleceptors (the sense of the outside world that we receive through our eyes, ears, and skin). This matchup provided her with a basis of support from which she could move in new ways, walk up and down her stairs comfortably, and, most happily of all, take her dog for walks.

As a result of her improved balance habits, Jennifer began to breathe much more easily, her jaw began to loosen as the muscles relaxed, and she stopped grinding her teeth at night. When I last saw Jennifer, not only was she balancing on the balls of her feet while turning her head from side to side, but she was also able to balance on one leg at a time.

● ● ●

14 AND 15. IS IT DIFFICULT FOR YOU TO JUMP?
IS IT DIFFICULT FOR YOU TO HOP ON ONE LEG?

To jump or hop, we must make sure that our limbs and trunk are coordinated. And to hop, we especially need better balance. These movements will improve many actions that also require good balance and coordination.

How to Transform Your Habits

First, while standing, just raise your heels from the floor and then lower them. Rather than lifting your whole body in the air, go up a small amount on the balls of your feet. You can do this slowly a few times, and then more quickly.

Not being able to hop well indicates balance difficulties. Stand near something you can hold on to—a counter or a wall—and simply stand on one leg. Can you maintain this position for ten seconds or so? Try the other leg. Some people start to feel faint because they stop breathing, so keep your jaw relaxed. Then, just as you "jumped" without leaving the floor, move your upper body up and down by simply raising and lowering the heel of one foot and then the other.

See the following lessons:

Lesson 2: Releasing the Hips into Pleasure
Lesson 6: Regaining Full Use of Your Neck
Lesson 8: The Middle of the Body: Expanding, Reaching, and Turning
Lesson 14: The Sitting and Turning Dance
Lesson 25: Freeing Stiff Hips and Knees
Lesson 26: Improving Balance
Lesson 29: Jumping to Discover Your Posture
Lesson 30: Hopping for Health

16. DO YOU KNOCK INTO THINGS AND GET BRUISES WITHOUT KNOWING HOW?

As we age, there is a decrease in the amount of what is called somato-sensory feedback from our muscles and joints to our brain. This can be especially true in our feet and lower extremities. Because many people live most of their life using only a small percentage of the body awareness available to them, it becomes more necessary, even critical, to improve body awareness as we age.

How to Transform Your Habits

Put a small piece of furniture, like a small chair or a big wastepaper basket, on one side of your door. Walk through your door, forward and then backward, without knocking into your door frame or kicking the piece of furniture.

How do you do it? Pretend you're dancing the tango and have to be precise. Feel how you organize your body when you have to think about it.

See the following lessons:

Lesson 1: Coordinating Your Neck and Eyes with Your Legs and Pelvis
Lesson 5: Rolling into Length Across Your Stomach
Lesson 6: Regaining Full Use of Your Neck
Lesson 7: A Simple Rolling Lesson
Lesson 14: The Sitting and Turning Dance
Lesson 15: Moving from the Chair to the Floor and Returning
Lesson 19: Finding the Two Halves of Your Body
Lesson 20: Crawling with Your Knees Up and Down
Lesson 21: Upright Kneeling
Lesson 25: Freeing Stiff Hips and Knees
Lesson 26: Improving Balance

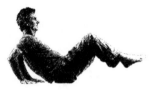

17. IS THERE A LACK OF SENSATION IN YOUR FEET AND LEGS, MAKING YOU FEEL INSECURE ABOUT YOUR BALANCE?

As we get older, the input from sensory receptors in our feet, ankles, and knees—from our lower extremities generally—diminishes. This is particularly true for people who do not get regular exercise.

How to Transform Your Habits

Spend some time sitting on the ground or in a chair and playing with your toes. Pull your toes in different directions. Make friends with your feet. Move the bones of your feet around with your hands. Then stand up and notice how large your feet feel.

See the following lessons:

Lesson 1: Coordinating Your Neck and Eyes with Your Legs and Pelvis
Lesson 2: Releasing the Hips into Pleasure

Lesson 6: Regaining Full Use of Your Neck
Lesson 9: Crossed-Arm, Crossed-Ankle Foot Lifting—Advanced Lying
   Lesson
Lesson 16: Jump-Sitting in a Chair
Advanced Variation on Lesson 16: Jump-Sitting on the Floor
Lesson 21: Upright Kneeling
Lesson 22: Through Crouching to Standing
Lesson 25: Freeing Stiff Hips and Knees
Lesson 27: The Ultimate Walking Lesson
Lesson 28: Standing on the Highest Point of the Hip
Lesson 29: Jumping to Discover Your Posture
Lesson 30: Hopping for Health

18. IS IT DIFFICULT FOR YOU TO WALK FORWARD AND BACKWARD SO SLOWLY THAT IT TAKES TEN SECONDS TO COMPLETE ONE STEP?

To walk very slowly forward or backward requires greater balancing skills than to stand on one leg or the other. When you balance on one leg, you tend to remain in a fixed position, but when you walk slowly forward and backward, your muscles are constantly changing, and so are the pressures through your joints. Your vestibular system must be more active than it is when holding your body in one position.

How to Transform Your Habits
Practice walking forward and backward slowly (about ten seconds for a step). Do this next to a wall for support if you are feeling unsure of yourself. As you become more comfortable and sure-footed, you will be able to walk backward faster with ease and your balance will improve walking forward.
   See the following lessons:

Lesson 1: Coordinating Your Neck and Eyes with Your Legs and Pelvis
Lesson 14: The Sitting and Turning Dance

● ● ●

I HOPE you find the movements suggested here useful. Remember, the best way to do the Change Your Age Program is to do it all from the beginning and not limit yourself to what you see as your habits. It's not so easy for us to have an accurate view of our own habits.

By relearning your habits, you will establish the basis for changing the fundamental organization of your movements and for changing your age for life.

CHAPTER SIX

CHANGE YOUR AGE FOR LIFE

I HOPE you have found that this program—the lessons in Chapter 3, the Change Your Age Mobility Survey, and the specialized routines outlined in Chapters 4 and 5—is a radical and useful way to begin or improve an exercise routine by expanding your body awareness. This program asks you to coordinate your brain as well as your body. I strongly encourage you to be inventive and experimental as you find ways to combine the lessons and real-life situations in which to use them.

But don't leave behind the lessons and insights you've learned here when you finish your exercise routine for the day or when you're not feeling any particular need for reenergizing or relaxing yourself. The awareness you gain from doing this program can be applied to your whole life and way of moving.

The basic principles of movement you've learned in doing the Change Your Age Program—increasing your body awareness, melting old movement habits while relearning new ways to move, activating your imagination, learning like a child through exploratory movement, breathing with your whole body, sensing your posture from the inside—should certainly be applied not just to your exercise routine but to your entire life. By listening to your body and using your mind to relearn how to move, you can improve your wellbeing beyond any measure of body strength, flexibility, or weight and truly change your age for life!

193

BODY AWARENESS

As discussed in this book, body awareness is needed to improve your exercise routine, but it can do so much more. Developing your body awareness helps you understand the relationships between different parts of your body. For example, your habitual ways of moving your legs affect the work of your shoulders, head, and neck, just as the way you tighten your neck, shoulders, and jaw affects your lower back, hips, and knees. If you can understand how you organize your body, you can reduce pain or eliminate painful movement and deal more effectively with the consequences of injury.

Sometimes the smallest adjustments, invisible to an outside observer, can alleviate discomfort you may have long ago accepted as a fact of aging. The greater body awareness nurtured by the Change Your Age Program can help you understand and improve not only how you move when you are exercising but also how you perform the ordinary tasks of life—driving through traffic, bending down or kneeling for yard work, loading a dishwasher, carrying a child, or hoisting a bag of groceries up on one hip.

I've had clients who thought they could no longer take adventure trips once they reached a certain age. They discovered that, with the same muscles, ligaments, and bones they'd always had, but exercising newfound body awareness, they could go on steep mountain hikes, go kayaking, or play tennis again.

Too often we pat ourselves on the back for exercising three times a week, getting our heart rate up, and building muscles and flexibility, but then ignore our bodies and the way we move when we finish working out. The Change Your Age Program asks more from you. It asks you to continue to be aware of your body beyond the gym or sports field and to use your brain to apply movement lessons to all the movements of your life, from the mundane (taking out the trash) to the extraordinary (sex).

DEVELOP HEALTHIER HABITS

With your newly honed body awareness, you can use the Change Your Age Program to become aware of lifelong bad habits and to figure out how to relearn certain movements and develop healthier habits going forward. Most of us form our habits at an early age, then become unaware of them. We might not notice our posture unless someone points out that we are slumped or until we feel a painful tightness in the back. Most of the time we don't forge a connection in our body-mind between, say, a painful way of stepping, as a result of an old ankle injury, and an overly tight bite and stiff neck, but in this program those are just the connections you need to make. Recognizing your habits and learning healthier ones is extremely important to improving your exercise routine, but doing so is also vital to bringing greater mobility into your everyday activities, including the ones you hope to keep performing in the future.

You may discover something magical as you reexamine your habits: Whatever you do and however you move, you can rely on the universal constants of ground forces and gravity, which can help you in everything you do. For example, if one of your legs feels weaker than the other when you're climbing stairs, you can address it by applying something you've learned here: how to observe yourself pushing down through your standing leg in order to lift your other leg. That simple principle can save you from feelings of weakness, imbalance, or incapacity. All it requires is a recognition of universal forces and the knowledge that you can transform your body intelligence to use those forces as friends. If you try using only your arms while lifting a weight, you may need to reorganize your body with some new habits by paying more attention to your balance and gravity and your connection to the ground. You may need to engage your legs and your back in the effort. Adjusting how you organize your body and your attention when you lift something can help you immeasurably, whether you are lifting weights at the gym or groceries out of the trunk.

Make sure you apply the new habits that improve your workout to your whole life and all of its movements.

IMAGINATION

One of our key tools in developing better movement habits and changing our age is our imagination. Often in these lessons you are asked to imagine a movement before performing it. It is tremendously useful to visualize every aspect of a movement, from how your shoulders are aligned in relation to your torso, to the view you will have as you turn your head, to how you look viewed from a different angle, to how and which body parts press against the floor, to how you shift your posture in preparation for a movement, to how you feel inside experiencing the movement. All of these images and more will fire your neurons, create new synaptic connections, and help you grow a new brain. With this "bigger," sharper mind, you can more easily perform the imagined movement. The mental dress rehearsal prepares your entire body to move when you ask it to.

You can apply the concept of imagining movement beyond the arena of sports. You will certainly find that visualization improves your workouts, especially when you are trying new routines, and your performance of repetitive athletic motions, like swinging a tennis racket or golf club, but using your imagination doesn't need to stop there. You can practice visualizing ordinary activities like brushing your teeth or hair, getting in and out of your car, or walking up and down stairs. In fact, visualization is a good way to foster greater body awareness in times when you aren't usually paying attention to what you are doing and to reinforce the healthier habits you are learning.

You might realize that you understand your movements and habits better than you thought you did, but that you have built a kind of wall around your exercise routine that has prevented you from applying the lessons learned there to your everyday movements.

USING EXPLORATORY MOVEMENTS TO LEARN

In combination with growing our brains through imagination, using exploratory movements to learn as we did when we were infants and children is extremely important in developing new habits and changing our age. You already know a lot of varied movements but may have lost or forgotten them as you've aged. By exploring and experimenting with novel movement, you can unlock the vault of your movement knowledge and solve the mystery of how to combine movements in spontaneous, new, and more functional ways.

In this program, you've been performing novel movements that aren't derived from the already existing systems familiar to many people from classes taught at gyms, like yoga and Pilates. Exercising in traditional ways, including walking and running, doesn't require that you learn new ways to move. Most exercise systems, in fact, require that you just repeat things you already know. By learning a novel movement, you can break away more easily from old, ingrained, unhealthy habits and develop new ones.

Like a baby rocking forward in an attempt to crawl or playing by placing his feet in a certain way that allows him to try standing, you can experiment with your body, exploring which ways of moving feel most natural or effective. Finding the best and easiest way to move when you are learning a new movement is a crucial lesson. Once learned, it can be applied to all everyday movements, whether the repetitive actions in a workout program or the unusual torquing and twisting we do when we turn around in the driver's seat to parallel-park a car or reach down to retrieve a fallen utensil.

By using your body to solve puzzles in movement, you are not only learning the practical physical effects of an exercise or habitual movement but also creating a new brain. You are forging new interconnections and encouraging the growth of new neurons in the same way we all did as infants and children when we played movement games with our bodies, like hopscotch and tag.

We need to reintroduce the way we learned movement as children to our adult lives. I want to encourage you to apply the same notion to movements you know so well that you could do them in your sleep. Experiment with finding different ways of getting out of your favorite chair, or play with three or four different ways of going up and down the stairs, or any other everyday activity. Not only will you gain greater body awareness and understanding of your habits, but you will also grow your brain and broaden the application of your new ways of moving from your workout sessions to your everyday activities.

BREATHING AND POSTURE

Before I leave you to integrate this program into your life, I want to reemphasize the new ways of thinking about the most fundamental elements of all of our movement—our breathing and our posture.

Even if you are not moving but are sitting in a chair or lying in bed, you are still organizing your body in motion as you automatically and involuntarily inhale and exhale. Understanding the muscle groups at work when you breathe can help you understand the basic physical state from which all your other movements emerge. If you breathe from your chest, for example, as people with anxiety issues often do, you may be restricting the movement of your ribs and tightening your head, neck, and shoulders, which can lead to greater difficulty in pivoting on a basketball court, turning to look behind you when walking down the street, or even just staying calm.

When you inhale, you use primarily the large group of muscles called the diaphragm. If your trunk—the muscles around your ribs, the muscles connecting your spine to your ribs, the muscles near your solar plexus, below your chest but above your navel—is tight, then you experience continual resistance to the act of inhaling. What's interesting is that when you exhale, a huge number of muscles in your trunk—about 60 muscles, some of them very large and strong—engage all at once. So if you inhale fully and blow out your air suddenly, you'll feel muscles in your abdominal wall, waist, back, and ribs all participating in the exhalation. Therefore, it's much easier to breathe out than to breathe in.

Addressing how you breathe while you move is the first step to improving how you move. And no movement leads to real improvement if you have to hold your breath to accomplish it.

Remember, as discussed earlier, good posture means preparing your body to execute the next movement you want to do. Your posture is so much more than a mechanical event. In your posture, you express your attitudes, your most basic emotions, the influences of your culture, and often your intentions. Your posture contains a story—the story of your life. It's both a biological phenomenon and a representation of the state of your body-mind. All your movements grow out of your posture, and what lends meaning to your movement and posture is your orientation. You have a posture, and you orient yourself to move toward or away from something. You might put on a posture hoping people will see you a certain way, and you might wear your most comfortable posture only when alone or with loved ones. You don't learn in order to move; you move in order to learn.

As you get older, remember that you will have acquired more skills and you can choose to pay more attention to how you are embodied. I hope the information you've gained from the Change Your Age Program will give you a longer, happier, and more adventuresome life.

Don't limit your newfound knowledge to when you are doing the lessons. Most of us don't have the time to spend an hour each day to stay in shape . . . nor do we need to. Bring all of the mundane, everyday activities you perform anyway into your practice. Choose to act with awareness, using your body's intelligence, every time you walk, drive, sit down, get up, bend, kneel, reach, twist, or turn. Think of the various distinctions you have encountered in these lessons as an alphabet of movement. You have learned the different letters that you can now begin to put together into words and sentences.

It may take a couple of weeks to learn the lessons and begin to see improvements in your mobility, but once you start, you will be able to achieve your goal of changing your age by ten or more years, and even better, you will then be at the point where you can set new goals and keep improving with age.

ABOUT THE AUTHOR

For forty years, Frank Wildman has been a leader of the "Movement Movement," showing people the hidden intelligence of their minds and bodies. His international instruction and mentoring have allowed thousands to move with greater freedom and regain a youthful state of painless ease and comfort.

His career began as a young performing artist, choreographer, and dancer. During his work with Anna Halprin's dance troupe in San Francisco, he met renowned physicist, engineer, and judo master Moshe Feldenkrais. Fascinated by Feldenkrais's perspective on human motion, Wildman went on to study with him for a decade while simultaneously acquiring degrees in physical education, biology, and somatic psychology. His work led to advances in physical therapy, which have been adopted internationally by hospitals, universities, physical and occupational therapists, and somatic psychologists.

Following Feldenkrais's death in 1984, Wildman set to work on building the future for the Feldenkrais Method®. With the goal of education being top priority, Wildman became the first educational director of a Feldenkrais Professional Training Program and guided the certification of a host of Feldenkrais practitioners and allied health professionals. As a president of the Feldenkrais Guild of North America, he helped develop and define the standards of practice that are the current international guidelines.

As educational director of The Feldenkrais Movement Institute, Dr. Wildman continues to draw interest in his programs from medical and educational professionals. He is a sought after speaker at seminars and symposia, where he's known for his dynamic teaching and visionary style of educating.

He has been called on to present for many prestigious health organizations, among them the American Society on Aging; the International and American Pain Societies; the International Congress of Physiotherapy; the American Fibromyalgia Council; the American Physical Therapy Association; the Canadian and Australian Physiotherapy Associations; the American Back Society; the International Federation for Orthopedic Manipulative Therapists; the International Council for Health and Physical Recreation, Sport and Dance and the Australian Institute for Sport.

Frank Wildman is the creator of an avalanche of educational materials in the form of audio and video courses as well as books. He is married and lives in Berkeley. He holds a private practice in Berkeley and also consults with individuals in New York, Australia, Japan, Italy, and Paris. For more information on Dr. Wildman and the various products available, please visit www.changeyourage.net.

OTHER EDUCATIONAL MATERIALS
BY FRANK WILDMAN

Books

Feldenkrais: The Busy Person's Guide to Easier Movement
Fibromyalgia: Relief from Chronic Muscle Pain
   (co-authored with Paul Davidson, MD)

CDs

"The Intelligent Body," 24-CD series
"Moving from Pain into Pleasure"
"Better Driving"
"Dealing with Back Pain"
"TMJ Lessons"

DVDs

"Improving with Age," 4-DVD series
"Your Brain as the Core of Strength and Stability," 2-volume DVD series

ACKNOWLEDGMENTS

THIS BOOK was created through the influence and inspiration provided by many people I feel close to. I'd first like to acknowledge my teacher and mentor, the greatest movement scientist of the twentieth century, Dr. Moshe Feldenkrais.

I had another book in mind entirely when I started this process, but then, through inspired discussions with my friend and colleague Paula Batson and the wonderful publishing strategist Janet Goldstein, who helped me shape the proposal, I realized how *Change Your Age* could be developed into an extremely useful book for many people. Thank you to both Janet and Paula, and especially to my agent Sarah Lazin, for helping to turn a cornucopia of ideas into a single book.

I would like to give my greatest thanks to Margarita Strmecki, my administrative assistant, whose tireless work ethic and positive attitude made it possible to complete this book.

Thank you to Renée Sedliar of Da Capo Press for keeping me on track and being a find of an editor. I also thank Chris Lambert in Australia, Chrish Kresge in Washington, D.C., and Dr. Sandy Rosenberg in San Francisco—all smart, caring friends and colleagues who kindly reviewed the book and gave hours of time and feedback.

I could not thank my wife, Viviana Diaz, enough for her critical thinking skills, editing contributions, and unwillingness to settle for anything less than the best.

Kudos to R. J. Muna, who supplied gorgeous photos and provided the challenge to write as well as he shoots, and to the models Carolyn Cavalier, Viviana Diaz, and Jeff Smith.

Thanks to my colleagues Dr. Jim Stephens for your much-needed research advice and support, Anastasi Siotas for your reframing, and Dwight Pargee and Frank Funk for your advice and tips.

Thank you, my dear friend Dr. Ken Dychtwald, for adding years of inspiration about the positive side of aging and for writing such a beautiful foreword to *Change Your Age*.

NOTES

1. K. Fabel and G. Kempermann, "Physical Activity and the Regulation of Neurogenesis in the Adult and Aging Brain," *Neuromolecular Medicine* (February 20, 2008).

2. P. E. Hartman-Stein and E. S. Potkanowicz, "Behavioral Determinants of Healthy Aging: Good News for the Baby Boomer Generation," *Online Journal Issues Nursing* 8, no. 2 (2003): 6.

3. C. W. Cotman and N. C. Berchtold, "Exercise: A Behavioral Intervention to Enhance Brain Health and Plasticity," *Trends in Neuroscience* 25, no. 6 (June 2002): 295–301.

4. Ibid.

5. J. D. Churchill, R. Galvez, S. Colcombe, R. A. Swain, A. F. Kramer, and W. T. Greenough, "Exercise, Experience, and the Aging Brain," *Neurobiological Aging* 23, no. 5 (September–October 2002): 941–955.

INDEX

p26
43
61 head turning at.
62 over contracting neck muscles

172 startle reflex